Up-to-Date Approach to Blood Gas Analysis – Clues to Diagnosis and Treatment

Edited by Özgür Karcıoğlu,
Canan Akman and Neslihan Ergün Süzer

Published in London, United Kingdom

Up-to-Date Approach to Blood Gas Analysis – Clues to Diagnosis and Treatment
http://dx.doi.org/10.5772/intechopen.1003490
Edited by Özgür Karcıoğlu, Canan Akman and Neslihan Ergün Süzer

Contributors

Ali Kashefi, Asieh Emami Nejad, Canan Akman, Erwin Michel Davila-Iniesta, Foivos Leonidas Mouzakis, Félix Gil-Carrasco, Jan Wilhelm Spillner, Johannes Greven, Khosrow Mottaghy, Lal Babu Khadka, Luis Niño-de-Rivera, Marjan Taherian, Mojtaba Ahmadlou, Mostafa Manian, Neslihan Ergün Süzer, Semin Turhan, Özgür Karcıoğlu

Notice

Statements and opinions expressed in the chapters are these of the individual contributors and not necessarily those of the editors or publisher. No responsibility is accepted for the accuracy of information contained in the published chapters. The publisher assumes no responsibility for any damage or injury to persons or property arising out of the use of any materials, instructions, methods or ideas contained in the book.

First published in London, United Kingdom, 2025 by IntechOpen
IntechOpen is the global imprint of INTECHOPEN LIMITED, registered in England and Wales, registration number: 11086078, 167-169 Great Portland Street, London, W1W 5PF, United Kingdom

For EU product safety concerns: IN TECH d.o.o., Prolaz Marije Krucifikse Kozulić 3, 51000 Rijeka, Croatia, info@intechopen.com or visit our website at intechopen.com.

British Library Cataloguing-in-Publication Data
A catalogue record for this book is available from the British Library

Up-to-Date Approach to Blood Gas Analysis – Clues to Diagnosis and Treatment
Edited by Özgür Karcıoğlu, Canan Akman and Neslihan Ergün Süzer
p. cm.
Print ISBN 978-0-85014-823-7
Online ISBN 978-0-85014-822-0
eBook (PDF) ISBN 978-0-85014-824-4

If disposing of this product, please recycle the paper responsibly.

We are IntechOpen,
the world's leading publisher of
Open Access books
Built by scientists, for scientists

7,500+
Open access books available

196,000+
International authors and editors

215M+
Downloads

Our authors are among the

156
Countries delivered to

Top 1%
most cited scientists

12.2%
Contributors from top 500 universities

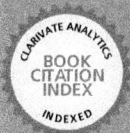

CLARIVATE ANALYTICS
BOOK
CITATION
INDEX
INDEXED

WEB OF SCIENCE™

Selection of our books indexed in the Book Citation Index
in Web of Science™ Core Collection (BKCI)

Interested in publishing with us?
Contact book.department@intechopen.com

Numbers displayed above are based on latest data collected.
For more information visit www.intechopen.com

Meet the editors

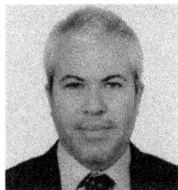

Dr. Özgür Karcıoğlu started residency in 1994 at Dokuz Eylul University Medical School, Department of Emergency Medicine. He completed the Fellowship Program in International Emergency Medicine at Pennsylvania State University in 2005. From 2005 to 2007, he served as the chairman of the department at DEU. He then led the Emergency Department at Bakirkoy Research and Training Hospital from 2007 to 2009, before joining Acıbadem University as a faculty member from 2009 to 2015. Currently, he is a full professor and chair at the Istanbul Education and Research Hospital in İstanbul. Dr. Karcıoğlu was a founder and board member of the Emergency Medical Association of Turkey from 2007 to 2009. Around 200 of his articles have been published in international journals, and he has contributed as an editor to five books, authoring 40 chapters. He also serves as a member of the editorial board for several journals and is an instructor for the American Heart Association-based Basic and Advanced Cardiac Life Support Course.

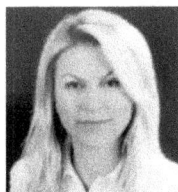

Associate Prof. Dr. Canan Akman completed her specialization at Hacettepe University Faculty of Medicine, Department of Emergency Medicine. Between 2012 and February 16, 2016, she worked as the First Emergency Medicine Specialist and Administrator at Kanuni Sultan Süleyman Training and Research Hospital in Istanbul. In 2014, she was awarded the title of Physician of the Year in Istanbul. She is actively involved in the toxicology, trauma, pediatric emergency, and geriatric working groups within the Emergency Medicine Association of Turkey (EMAT). Dr. Akman was appointed as an Associate Professor in 2021. Since September 23, 2021, she has been serving as an Education Coordinator and Faculty Board Member at Çanakkale Onsekiz Mart University, while continuing her role as Assistant Medical Director. In addition, she completed a master's degree in Medical Education at Çanakkale Onsekiz Mart University Institute of Educational Sciences in 2021. Currently, she is affiliated with the Hindawi Emergency Medicine Journal. To date, she has published 63 articles and authored 13 books.

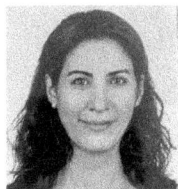

Assistant Prof. Dr. Neslihan Ergün Süzer started her specialization in 2010 at the Istanbul Training and Research Hospital Emergency Medicine Clinic. She served as the Emergency Department Physician in charge from 2015 to 2017 and continued as an Emergency Department Physician from 2017 to 2023 at Kocaeli Gebze Fatih State Hospital. In 2023, she began working at Kocaeli Darıca Farabi Training and Research Hospital, where she continues her role. Dr. Süzer is an official Turkish Emergency Medicine Association member and ATUDER (Emergency Medicine Specialists Association) member. She has published 9 articles in international journals and 2 in national journals, authored 5 book chapters, and served as an editor for 1 book. She has obtained various certifications from Emergency Medicine Associations, including

Basic and Advanced Ultrasound, Mechanical Ventilator Use, Statistics, and Critical Patient Care. Additionally, she has delivered 5 oral presentations at congresses—4 at the international level and 1 at the national level. Her doctoral thesis focuses on arterial blood gas values in the preoxygenation phase of emergency department patients for whom intubation decisions were made using the rapid sequence intubation protocol.

Contents

Preface

Analysis of arterial blood gases (ABG) plays an important role in the evaluation of critical diseases and in determining the etiology and severity of diseases. Experimental and mathematical methods for assessing acid-base balance and ventilation were developed in the last century.

In ABG analysis, two main functions of respiration, namely ventilation and oxygenation, are examined. Measurements of oxygen (PaO2) and CO2 partial pressures (PaCO2), oxygen saturation (SaO2), pH, and HCO3 values in arterial blood are performed by ABG analysis to evaluate acid-base balance and respiratory status. On the other hand, glucose, electrolyte, kidney functions, bilirubin and hemoglobin levels can also be checked in ABG analysis and information about the metabolic status can be elicited with the devices developed in recent years.

Evaluation of ABG is a valuable asset in providing information about the severity of the disease in clinical follow-up. Indications for ABG analysis can be summarized as follows: Diagnosis and follow-up of metabolic and respiratory acidosis and alkalosis, recognition of the type of respiratory failure, information on the effectiveness of the treatment provided, indication and follow-up of O2 therapy, and revealing the cause of dyspnea.

Blood gas analysis is one of modern medicine's most essential diagnostic tools, providing critical information about patients' oxygenation, ventilation, and acid-base balance. With a broad range of applications, from emergency departments to intensive care units, from internal medicine and surgical clinics to anesthesia practice, this analysis plays a vital role in patient management when interpreted correctly.

With advancing technology and evolving treatment approaches, blood gas analysis remains an indispensable tool for healthcare professionals. Therefore, this book project is intended to reveal the indications and drawbacks of ABG and to draw the boundaries of this method in contemporary medicine.

This book has been prepared for all physicians and healthcare professionals who wish to understand blood gas analysis better and integrate it into their clinical practice. It covers fundamental physiological principles and thoroughly examines conditions such as acidosis, alkalosis, respiratory and metabolic disorders, hypoxemia, and hypercapnia. Additionally, it addresses current topics such as pre- and post-intubation blood gas management, toxic alcohols and their relation with metabolic status and blood gases, mechanical ventilation optimization, and the role of blood gas analysis in critical patient monitoring. We hope this book will be a valuable resource for all healthcare providers seeking to enhance their knowledge and skills in blood gas analysis and related clinical issues.

Sincerely,

Özgür Karcıoğlu, M.D.
Professor,
Istanbul Education and Research Hospital,
University of Health Sciences,
Istanbul, Türkiye

Canan Akman, M.D.
Associate Professor,
Faculty of Medicine,
Department of Emergency Medicine,
Canakkale Onsekiz Mart Univeristy,
Canakkale, Türkiye

Dr. Neslihan Ergün Süzer
Assistant Professor,
Kocaeli Darıca Farabi Training and Research Hospital,
Health Sciences University,
Kocaeli, Türkiye

Chapter 1

Introductory Chapter: Arterial Blood Gases – Canary in the Mine?

Özgür Karcıoğlu, Canan Akman and Neslihan Ergün Süzer

1. Introduction

A woman in her sixties was brought to the ED with a history of heart failure for 8 years and diabetes for 26 years. She was found to have dyspnea, tachypnea, and tachycardia. Her complaints have worsened progressively over the past 3 to 4 days, especially when she lies down. She says that she had been fighting a cold 2 weeks ago, and a greenish sputum persisted thereafter. She appears anxious and agitated but denies chest pain, nausea, vomiting, diaphoresis, or fever. She is a smoker with 60 packs/years (40 years and 1.5 packs of cigarettes a day). She has been diagnosed with bronchitis several times and was hospitalized 3 years ago with pneumonia. She has gained around four kilograms over the last months. Her respiratory rate was 32 bpm, heart rate 116 bpm, SaO2 87% at 4 L/min O2 via nasal cannula on the ambulance. High-flow nasal cannula oxygen therapy increased SaO2 to 93% in the ED.

On the complete blood count, she has increased her leukocyte count 12.400 10^9/L. Blood glucose is 270 mg/dL and serum creatinine is 1.6 mg/dL. Arterial blood gas values turns out to be pH 7.33, PaO2 88 mmHg and PaCO2 52 mmHg on the initial examination on room air.

Highlight: Almost everyday, emergency physicians encounter patients such as this lady, in whom many factors contribute to the cause of the ED visit and complicate the clinical picture. Routine investigations help enlighten the differential diagnosis, but oxygenation and ventilation can be obscured after these. Respiratory failure and clinical deterioration despite treatment, can be overlooked in the absence of arterial blood gases.

2. Role of arterial blood gases (ABG) in evaluation of critical patients

ABG analysis has an important role in the assessment of critical diseases and in determining the etiology and severity of many entities. ABG is useful in the management of various respiratory and metabolic disturbances.

Measurement of oxygen (PaO2) and carbon dioxide partial pressures (PaCO2), oxygen saturation (SaO2), pH and bicarbonate values in arterial blood is performed by ABG analysis in the evaluation of acid-base and respiratory balances [1].

Two basic functions of respiration are examined in blood gas analysis: ventilation and oxygenation. Multiple pathological entities can be recognized in critically ill patients using analysis of the pH, PaO2, PaCO2, and SaO2, and comparing it to measured serum bicarbonate [2]. With the devices developed in recent years, glucose, electrolyte, kidney functions, bilirubin, and hemoglobin levels can be examined in the ABG analysis and information about the metabolic status can also be obtained. **Table 1** gives a summary of ingredients of ABG analysis to consider in routine practice.

Indications of ABG analysis include conditions such as respiratory failure, ventilation-perfusion mismatch, metabolic acidosis or alkalosis, and acute respiratory diseases are typical indications for the use of ABG. Indications for ABG analysis can be summarized as follows:

- Diagnosis and follow-up of metabolic and respiratory acidosis and alkalosis

- Determining the type of respiratory failure

- Evaluation of the effectiveness of the given treatment

- Indication and follow-up of oxygen therapy

Variable	Explanation	Pathological value thresholds
pH	Used to determine the H+ status of the blood. It shows that the patient is in acidosis or alkalosis, but it is not possible to understand the type only by pH. Normal values are between 7.35 and 7.45.	pH >7.45 = Alkalosis pH <7.35 = Acidosis
Partial Arterial Oxygen Pressure (PaO2):	The partial pressure of oxygen in arterial blood which is used to evaluate oxygenation. Normal values are 80–100 mmHg.	"mild hypoxemia" if between 60 and 79 mmHg "moderate hypoxemia" if it is between 40 and 59 mmHg "severe hypoxemia" if below 40 mmHg
Oxygen saturation (SaO2)	The oxygen saturation level of hemoglobin. Normal values are 95–100%.	
Partial Arterial Carbon Dioxide Pressure (PaCO2)	It is the partial pressure of carbon dioxide in arterial blood. It is an indicator of alveolar ventilation. Normal values are 35–45 mmHg.	pCO2 > 45 = Acidosis pCO2 < 35 = Alkalosis
Bicarbonate (HCO3–)	It is the serum concentration of bicarbonate ion. It is an important buffer in the blood and is used to evaluate the metabolic component of acid-base balance. Normally it is 22–26 mEq/L.	Increased values of actual bicarbonate indicate metabolic alkalosis, and decreased values indicate metabolic acidosis. HCO3 > 26 = Alkalosis HCO3 < 22 = Acidosis
Base excess (BE)	The amount of acid or base required to maintain the pH of fully oxygenated blood to 7.40 at 37°C and 40 mmHg pCO2; It is an indicator of metabolic status. Normal values of BE vary between −3 and + 3.	BE<3 = metabolic acidosis, BE > + 3 = metabolic alkalosis
Alveolar-Arterial Oxygen Gradient (p(A-a)O2)	The difference between alveolar and arterial pO2 levels. It gives general information about the gas exchange function of the lungs. Normally, p(A-a)O2 is 5 mmHg, but it increases with age, with an increase of 4 mmHg for every 10 years after the age of 20.	

Table 1.
Components of arterial blood gas analysis to take into account in the clinical setting.

- Sudden-onset and unexplained dyspnea

- Cardiac arrest situations and the effect of procedures including CPR or post-ROSC states

Clinical estimates about oxygenation status is mostly erroneous and have poor prognostic power in the clinical setting. For example, one of the most important clinical signs, cyanosis is affected by the level of hemoglobin, skin color, perfusion and lighting status. In most circumstances, ABG and SpO2 offer an accurate measurement of oxygenation to guide diagnosis and management in the acute setting.

Likewise, SaO2 and SpO2 have their inherent deficiencies to demonstrate ventilatory function. An important criterion to oversee deterioration in the patient is to be informed on rising PaCO2 in respiratory failure or respiratory arrest. SaO2 and SpO2 heralds this kind of worsening status considerably lately in a sedated patient when consciousness is depressed or periarrest situations [3].

Sampling for ABG analysis triggers unwelcome experiences for patients. In addition, the procedure is accompanied by complications like arterial injury, thrombosis, air or clotted-blood embolism, arterial occlusion, hematoma, aneurysm formation, and reflex sympathetic dystrophy [4].

3. Interpretation of blood gases

Blood gas evaluation in clinical follow-up is a valuable tool that provides information on the severity of the disease. PaO2 represents oxygenation, and PaCO2 shows alveolar ventilation. The clinician must be aware of the normal values in the examination of ABG, which has a pivotal place in the clinical approach. The patient's clinical condition and other laboratory findings should also be taken into consideration in the clinical decision-making process in addition to ABG findings.

Blood gas measuring devices directly measure pH and PCO2 and calculate bicarbonate using the Henderson-Hasselbach equation.

$$pH = 6.1 + \log([HCO3]/[0.03xPCO2]). \tag{1}$$

PaO2 and PaCO2 give insight for gas exchange, while pH, PaCO2, and HCO3 are the parameters used to evaluate the acid-base status [1]. Of note is that the alveolar-arterial oxygen gradient is beneficial as a surrogate of pulmonary gas exchange, which can be abnormal in patients with a ventilation-perfusion mismatch [5].

In addition to evaluation of the patients' ventilatory, respiratory, and acid-base status, analysis of ABG is useful for assessment of the response to modes of treatment and monitoring the degree and progression of cardiopulmonary disease processes [6, 7]. Of note, incompatible or discrepant values are a potential drawback of the analysis of ABG; therefore, clinicians should strive to eliminate potential sources of error [8].

Finally, it should be taken into account that ABG results may be inaccurate due to laboratory errors and errors during sample collection. Interpretation of the ABG findings allows evaluation of the severity of disturbances, whether the imbalances are acute or chronic, and whether the primary disorder is primarily metabolic or respiratory [9].

4. Summary

ABG evaluates the physiological functions of the respiratory system, acid-base balance, and oxygen-carrying capacity through a blood gas analysis taken from an arterial blood sample, in this way. It plays a pivotal role in the evaluation of patients with critical diseases. In most clinical scenarios, PaO2 is examined to assess oxygenation, while PaCO2 is examined to evaluate ventilation. P(A-a)O2 is calculated to evaluate gas exchange. Conditions such as respiratory failure, ventilation-perfusion mismatch, metabolic acidosis or alkalosis, and acute respiratory diseases are accepted indications for the use of ABG.

Acid-base balance gains priority in most critical patients to intervene before correcting secondary problems. ABG interpretations prevent unnecessary use of imaging modalities and medications. Therefore, the patient's clinical condition and other laboratory findings should always be taken into consideration in the clinical decision-making process.

Funding source

None.

Conflict of interest

None.

Author details

Özgür Karcıoğlu[1*], Canan Akman[2] and Neslihan Ergün Süzer[3]

1 Department of Emergency Medicine, Istanbul Education and Research Hospital, University of Health Sciences, Istanbul, Turkey

2 Department of Emergency Medicine, Canakkale Onsekiz Mart University, Canakkale, Turkey

3 Department of Emergency Medicine, Darica Farabi Education and Research Hospital, Kocaeli, Turkey

*Address all correspondence to: okarcioglu@gmail.com

IntechOpen

References

[1] Sarnaik AP, Heidemann SM. Respiratory pathophysiology and regulation. In: Behrman RE, Kliegman RM, Jenson HB, editors. Nelson Textbook of Pediatrics. 18th ed. Philadelphia: WB Saunders Company; 2007. pp. 1719-1726

[2] Gattinoni L, Pesenti A, Matthay M. Understanding blood gas analysis. Intensive Care Medicine. 2018;**44**(1):91-93

[3] Sivilotti M, Messenger D, Vlymen J. A comparative evaluation of capnometry versus pulse oximetry during procedural sedation and analgesia on room air. Canadian Journal of Emergency Medical Care. 2010;**12**:397-404

[4] Prasad H, Vempalli N, Agrawal N, et al. Correlation and agreement between arterial and venous blood gas analysis in patients with hypotension-an emergency department-based cross-sectional study. International Journal of Emergency Medicine. 2023;**16**(1):18. DOI: 10.1186/s12245-023-00486-0

[5] Hopkins SR. Ventilation/perfusion relationships and gas exchange: Measurement approaches. Comprehensive Physiology. 2020;**10**(3):1155-1205

[6] Castro D, Patil SM, Zubair M, Keenaghan M. Arterial blood gas. In: StatPearls [Internet]. Treasure Island (FL): StatPearls Publishing; 2024

[7] Davis MD, Walsh BK, Sittig SE, Restrepo RD. AARC clinical practice guideline: Blood gas analysis and hemoximetry: 2013. Respiratory Care. 2013;**58**(10):1694-1703

[8] Cowley NJ, Owen A, Bion JF. Interpreting arterial blood gas results. BMJ. 2013;**346**:f16

[9] Rogers KM, McCutcheon K. Four steps to interpreting arterial blood gases. Journal of Perioperative Practice. 2015;**25**(3):46-52

Chapter 2

Blood Gas Analyzers and Methodology

Marjan Taherian, Mojtaba Ahmadlou, Asieh Emami Nejad and Mostafa Manian

Abstract

The basic electrochemical techniques required for blood gas analysis were first introduced in the 1890s, leading to the development of arterial blood gas (ABG) analyzers that became clinically available in the 1950s. Modern blood gas analyzers utilize various electrodes to measure parameters such as partial pressures of arterial oxygen (PaO2), partial pressures of arterial carbon dioxide (PaCO2), and pH, making them vital diagnostic tools in healthcare settings. This chapter discusses the technical aspects of blood gas analysis, including the equipment and methods used to measure blood gases, as well as the differences between bench-top laboratory analyzers and portable patient-side analyzers. The importance of point-of-care testing (POCT) is highlighted, emphasizing its role in providing immediate laboratory results that enhance clinical decision-making, particularly in emergency and critical care situations. The analysis of blood gases, electrolytes, and metabolites is crucial for understanding patients' respiratory, circulatory, and metabolic conditions, ultimately improving patient outcomes through rapid and accurate testing.

Keywords: blood gas analyzers, arterial blood gas (ABG), partial pressure of arterial oxygen (PaO2), partial pressure of arterial carbon dioxide (PaCO2), point-of-care testing (POCT), acid-base status, oxygen saturation (SaO2)

1. Introduction

The basic electrochemical techniques required for blood gas analysis were first represented in the 1890s. The invention of electrodes to measure partial pressure of arterial oxygen (PaO2) by Clark, and partial pressure of arterial carbon dioxide (PaCO2) by Stowe, led to the development of arterial blood gas analyzers that became clinically available in the 1950s. ABGs were considered the most valuable laboratory examination in the 1960s [1]. Modern blood gas analyzers contain a Clark electrode for measuring the PaO2, a Stow-Severinghaus electrode for measuring the PaCO2, and a glass electrode for measuring pH [2]. Now, an arterial blood gas (ABG) machine is a vital diagnostic tool routinely used in healthcare settings to measure gases and various parameters in arterial blood, providing crucial data on oxygenation, respiration, and metabolic status. This equipment can be situated at the point of care of the patient and operated by laboratory staff or trained medical professionals.

IntechOpen

This important instrument comes in many varieties, each designed for specific clinical needs, ranging from basic models used in small clinics to advanced systems used in hospitals. In this chapter, we discuss the technical aspects of blood gas analysis and cover the equipment and methods used to measure blood gases.

2. Overview of blood gas analyzers

Blood gas analyzer is a commonly used diagnostic instrument to measure or calculate the partial pressures of blood gas, acid-base status, various electrolytes, and metabolites. The results provide valuable information that enables clinicians to interpret and understand the respiratory, circulatory, and metabolic conditions of patients [3]. This equipment is available in various sizes and weights and is usually divided into two types: bench-top laboratory analyzers and portable patient-side analyzers.

Bench-top analyzers are not usually portable and are often located in diagnostic laboratories, although newer models are significantly smaller and lighter than earlier models. Samples need to be transported to a lab to be analyzed with them; thus, it may take a long time. An example of a bench-top analyzer is the Nova Biomedical Critical Care Xpress Analyzer (Nova CCX; Nova Biomedical, Waltham, MA, USA), which provides reliable and accurate results [4]. Bench-top analyzers incorporate multi-use sensors with separate packages for reagents and quality control. Newer analyzers have replaced individual sensors and instead have sensor cards to facilitate regular maintenance. These sensor cards are supposed to last around 28–30 days, after which a new card is installed, allowing to replace all the sensors at once. These types of analyzers are more cost-effective and, like portable analyzers, require very small blood samples [5, 6].

Portable analyzers are ideal for patient-side or "point of care", allowing sample analysis at the patient's location, thereby eliminating turnaround time and time-to-treatment. These types of analyzers, including i-STAT (Abbott Point of Care Inc., Princeton, NJ, USA) and Enterprise Point-of-Care (EPOC) (Epocal Inc., Ottawa, ON, Canada), incorporate a single-use cartridge system containing the electrochemical sensors and calibration solution required in the analysis. The use of a disposable cartridge significantly reduces the need for maintenance and calibration of the analyzer hardware, as well as avoids the waste of time spent removing unwanted blood clots in a bench-top analyzer. Cartridges vary according to the composition of measured analytes so that some cartridges can measure up to 15 various analytes. Portable analyzers also make it possible to provide values easily and accurately even when used by non-specialist operators. When the cartridge is inserted into the handheld analyzer, it calibrates itself and brings the cartridge to a suitable temperature, so the operator only needs to enter the blood sample when the device is ready. The blood sample required for most of these models is very small, often around 95–97 microliters of blood or 2–3 drops. Despite these advantages, running large numbers of specimens with an individual sample cartridge-based analyzer is more expensive than with a bench-top analyzer [7, 8]. However, portability, minimal maintenance, and ease of use required make these analyzers strong contenders at the point of care.

3. Point-of-care testing (POCT)

Point-of-care testing (POCT) allows clinicians to overcome the barrier to accessing laboratory results in many ways and provides immediate availability of relevant laboratory tests that are useful in clinical decision-making. POCT can provide opportunities to expand patient care services and generate revenue [6].

The availability of POCT in the operating room, post-operative intensive care units (ICU), emergency department (ED), and pre-hospital transport systems (ambulance) reduces the time wasted in delivering samples to diagnostic laboratories or referral facilities that can delay appropriate treatment. Tissue oxygenation, ventilation, and acid-base status are the most vital parameters in the management of critically ill patients admitted in these emergency situations. Management strategies in these life-threatening situations depend heavily on rapid blood gas analysis. The development of POCT equipment with immediate blood gas analysis is essential in these conditions to optimize oxygenation and ventilation. As sudden physiological changes can occur in an anesthetized patient, immediate identification and treatment of problems can improve patient safety [9, 10]. There is accumulating evidence that point-of-care blood gas testing with rapid results (analysis typically takes 1–5 minutes) allows immediate interpretation and enables prompt implementation of targeted treatment plans, leading to reduced therapeutic turnaround time, and eventually improving patient outcomes [11, 12]. Studies have also indicated that these rapid results lead to a faster decision time compared to results from central laboratory testing and subsequent improvement of management strategies, thus reducing morbidity [13–15]. In addition, POCT significantly reduces the amount of blood required to measure parameters such as blood gases, electrolytes, glucose, lactates, and hemoglobin/hematocrit [9].

Although there are still debates among laboratories, clinicians, and administrators regarding the cost and implementation of POCT technology relative to conventional laboratory testing, and the fact that POCT for certain blood gases and electrolytes may not entirely supplant laboratory testing, it significantly alters the clinical practice paradigm for emergency and critical care physicians.

4. Point-of-care testing (POCT) in the diagnosis and management

Respiratory failure is a syndrome where the respiratory system fails to perform its gas exchange functions, leading to hypoxemia or hypercapnia. Examples include conditions like diabetic ketoacidosis (DKA) [16]. In DKA, the respiratory system can suffer from failure when the body tries to correct the acid-base balance, leading to potential complications and even death if prompt recognition and management are not taken [16].

POCT diagnostic systems can play a crucial role in the rapid diagnosis and management of respiratory failure by providing quick analysis time and high sensitivity. For example, POCT systems can measure biomarkers such as arterial blood gases and lactate levels to assess the severity of respiratory failure and guide appropriate treatment [17].

COPD is characterized by obstructed airflow due to chronic inflammation, making it difficult for individuals to exhale air efficiently. As a result, the alveoli do not get fully deflated, leading to increased dead space, which causes type 1 respiratory failure [16, 18, 19]. POCT diagnostic systems can aid in the diagnosis and management of COPD by providing rapid test results for assessing lung function, such as measuring arterial blood gases, which is crucial for determining the severity of COPD exacerbations and guiding treatment decisions [17, 20].

In the DKA condition, the body produces an excessive amount of ketone bodies as a result of insulin deficiency or insulin resistance, leading to metabolic acidosis.

This acid-base imbalance can cause altered breathing patterns, and increased ventilation attempts can exacerbate respiratory failure [21, 22]. In Addition, POCT systems can be valuable in the early diagnosis and management of DKA by measuring blood glucose and ketone levels, allowing for prompt initiation of treatment and monitoring of response to therapy. This is especially important in settings where immediate access to central laboratories may be limited [17].

Ethylene glycol ingestion leads to metabolic acidosis due to its metabolism into toxic byproducts such as oxalic acid, glycolic acid, and lactic acid. The increased acid production can cause a large anion gap and respiratory failure due to the body's compensatory mechanisms [23, 24]. Furthermore, POCT diagnostic systems can assist in the timely diagnosis and management of ethylene glycol poisoning by measuring specific biomarkers such as blood glucose, electrolytes, and toxic metabolites, enabling rapid intervention and treatment to prevent severe complications [17].

The reliability of POCT in the diagnosis and management of specific diseases such as respiratory failure, COPD, DKA, and ethylene glycol poisoning can be variable. For example, in the case of DKA, arterial blood gas analysis is essential for detecting respiratory failure, while in COPD, POCT may be more reliable for assessing oxygenation and acid-base status. Therefore, the use of POCT in these conditions should be carefully evaluated and tailored to the specific diagnostic and management needs of each disease [16]. Each condition presents unique challenges and considerations for POCT, including the need for accurate and timely results to guide clinical decisions. POCT can be valuable in providing rapid assessments of ABGs, electrolytes, and toxic substances, but it is important to consider the potential limitations, such as accuracy and precision, when interpreting results for these particular conditions. Additionally, the impact of technical issues with POCT devices on the reliability of results should be thoroughly discussed to provide a comprehensive overview of the subject [18].

For COPD, DKA, and ethylene glycol poisoning, the data for pH, PaCO2, PaO2, and HCO3 levels vary based on the specific disease and its stage or severity. In COPD, patients commonly present with elevated PaCO2 levels and decreased PaO2 levels due to impaired gas exchange, along with respiratory acidosis and elevated bicarbonate levels as compensatory mechanisms. When someone has DKA, they usually have metabolic acidosis (lower bicarbonate levels) and compensatory respiratory alkalosis (higher PaCO2 levels). The level of compensation depends on how bad the metabolic acidosis is. For ethylene glycol poisoning, metabolic acidosis with an increased anion gap and decreased bicarbonate levels is commonly observed, with variable respiratory compensation. Depending on the severity of poisoning, patients may exhibit varied PaCO2 and PaO2 levels due to respiratory compensation and potential secondary respiratory failure. It is important to note that these values can vary based on individual patient characteristics and the specific stage or severity of the disease [16].

Also, a previous study has provided insight into the ABG parameters associated with some neuromuscular diseases, aiding in the comparison and understanding of ABG abnormalities in intensive care unit patients with neuromuscular versus non-neuromuscular acute respiratory failure. It includes data for pH, PaCO2, PaO2, and HCO3 levels. Each disease, such as Myasthenia gravis and Guillain-Barré syndrome, is listed with the median values and interquartile ranges (IQR) for these ABG parameters. For example, for Myasthenia gravis, the median pH is 7.39 with an IQR of 7.32–7.4, the median PaCO2 is 39 with an IQR of 34.5–43.8, the median PaO2 is 88.1 with an IQR of 76.4–127.4, and the median HCO3 is 23.7 with an IQR of 19.3–26.3 [18]. These values can be measured through POCT diagnostic systems, providing rapid assessment and guiding treatment decisions in specific clinical settings [17].

On the other hand, POCT systems are essential for delivering rapid diagnostic results, facilitating timely on-site diagnosis and treatment. Essential characteristics of contemporary POCT diagnostic systems encompass rapid analysis time and elevated sensitivity, utilizing a sample-to-answer format. Microfluidic lab-on-a-chip technologies represent a promising solution for meeting the requirements of POCT. Microfluidic lab-on-a-chip technologies represent effective solutions by miniaturizing and integrating the majority of functional modules utilized in central laboratories into a compact chip [17, 20].

Furthermore, POCT systems identify specific biomarkers derived from proteins, cells, nucleic acids, metabolites, and other sources. The advancements in POCT technologies utilizing microfluidic lab-on-a-chip technologies have been emphasized, showcasing successful immunoassay POCT systems like the Triage cartridge and various other lab-on-a-chip systems for protein biomarker detection [25]. The Alere Triage system stands out as one of the most commercially successful immunoassay point-of-care testing systems. The Triage cartridge utilizes a working principle similar to that of lateral-flow assays, wherein target antigens in a sample initially bind to detection antibodies that are labeled with gold colloids. Previous studies have demonstrated the potential of microfluidic lab-on-a-chip technologies in delivering rapid analysis times and accomplishing complex diagnostic assays in a sample-to-answer format [17, 26].

These examples highlight the potential of POCT diagnostic systems in addressing the diagnostic and management needs of various medical conditions, especially in settings where immediate access to central laboratories and trained personnel may be limited [17, 26].

Taken together, POCT diagnostic systems are being developed in the world and have unique requirements for these systems, including the need for battery or solar power operation, stable reagents at high temperatures, and robustness for transport in resource-limited environments. It is of considerable importance [26]. Thus, at the outset of developing POCT diagnostic systems, it is essential to thoroughly evaluate the requirements for the intended objectives and performance criteria.

5. Principles of operation

Operation with a traditional analyzer begins with the operator providing a blood sample into the sample probe, which draws the blood sample with a peristaltic pump and loads the chamber with a specified amount of blood. The blood sample is then left in the chamber long enough to complete the measuring procedure. After that, the pump pushes the sample to waste. Automated blood gas analyzers are generally used to analyze blood gas samples, with results available within 10 to 15 minutes [27]. Common analyzers directly and indirectly determine several major areas of measurement:

5.1 Acid-base status

Analyzers indicate the acid-base balance by measuring two primary components, including PaCO2 and pH. pH is determined as the negative logarithm of H^+ activity in blood that can be affected by pCO2 function, and regulation of the body's pH level can greatly affect changes in pCO2.

5.1.1 pH

pH is determined as the negative logarithm of hydrogen ion (H^+) concentration (moles per liter) present in the blood, indicating the acidity or alkalinity of a blood sample. Blood pH is precisely maintained in the range of about 7.35–7.45 (usually 7.40), via different mechanisms involving the lungs, kidneys, and buffer systems [28, 29].

The blood carries carbon dioxide (CO_2), as a waste product of metabolism, to the lungs, where it is exhaled. As CO_2 combines with water to produce carbonic acid, the accumulation of CO_2 in the blood leads to increased acidity (decrease in the blood pH). The amount of carbon dioxide is controlled by adjusting the speed and depth of breathing (ventilation), thereby, the lungs are able to regulate the blood pH. Blood pH increases with faster and deeper breathing, increasing the amount of exhaled CO_2, while the decrease in ventilation and increase in pCO_2 leads to a decrease in blood pH. In addition, the kidneys are able to affect blood pH by regulating the rate of H^+ excretion. The chemical buffer systems, mainly carbonic acid (a weak acid formed from the CO_2 dissolved in blood) and bicarbonate ions (the corresponding weak base), are further involved in controlling blood pH.

Analyzers indicate the pH of the blood samples using a pH-measuring electrode and a reference electrode, known as the Sanz electrode [30]. The measuring electrode comprises silver-silver chloride and is encased in a pH-stabilized solution, enclosed by an $H+$ -sensitive glass membrane that allows the sample to transit. The resultant differential in $H+$ concentration across the membrane alters the voltage recorded by the electrode. The reference electrode consists of silver-silver chloride or calomel (mercury chloride) immersed in a saturated potassium chloride solution, producing a stable voltage. The voltage is compared to that produced at the measuring electrode when the sample transits through. The disparity between these voltages is transformed and displayed as the pH of the sample [31].

5.1.2 pCO2

Partial pressure is defined as the pressure exerted by a single gas in a mixture of gases or in a liquid and is calculated by multiplying the ratio of this gas by the total absolute pressure of the sample [32]. CO_2 is transported throughout the body in various forms, including a plasma-soluble molecular form, bound to hemoglobin, or most abundantly as a bicarbonate ion. CO_2 and oxygen balance the loading and unloading of each other onto hemoglobin. The binding of CO_2 to hemoglobin increases oxygen depletion (Bohr effect), while the binding of oxygen to hemoglobin (oxygenation of blood in the lungs) increases the removal of CO_2 (Haldane effect) [33]. The PCO_2 in a blood sample is assessed with a modified pH electrode known as the Severinghaus electrode. This electrode employs a silver-silver chloride reference electrode alongside a pH-measuring electrode. The measuring electrode is situated within a bicarbonate solution encased by a thin plastic barrier that permits CO_2 permeability while being impermeable to water, electrolytic solutes, and hydrogen ions. Upon diffusion of CO_2 across the membrane, it interacts with the bicarbonate solution, resulting in the formation of carbonic acid and subsequently $H+$ ions. This reaction alters the pH detected by the glass electrode, in the same manner as in the pH electrode [34]. The $PaCO_2$ value is normally measured in the range of 35–45 mm Hg.

5.2 Oxygen status

Analyzers measure the PaO2 in arterial blood, or the amount of oxygen gas in the whole blood.

5.2.1 pO2

Determination of pO2 reflects the uptake of oxygen in the body. PO2 is measured by a Clark electrode that consists of a silver-silver chloride anode and a centrally located platinum cathode [35]. This electrode is separated from the sample by an O2-permeable membrane. The cathode has a voltage potential of 0.7 V and, when exposed to oxygen, produces a current that draws electrons from the anode toward the cathode, reducing the oxygen. For each mole of oxygen, four electrons are drawn to the cathode. According to the reaction:

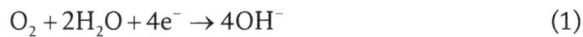

$$O_2 + 2H_2O + 4e^- \rightarrow 4OH^- \tag{1}$$

The silver is then oxidized and ionized at the anode to form silver chloride.

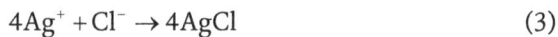

$$4\,Ag \rightarrow 4Ag^+ + 4e^- \tag{2}$$

$$4Ag^+ + Cl^- \rightarrow 4AgCl \tag{3}$$

The current produced by these reactions is proportional to the pO2 present in the sample [31]. The normal value of PaO2 is 75–100 mm Hg.

Furthermore, the modern blood gas analyzer enables to measure additional parameters by combining the results of various electrodes and applied calculations, for instance, measuring blood hemoglobin or the ability of oxygen to bind to this molecule. Current blood gas analyzers now have further Co-oximetry measurements to better evaluate hemodynamic values [36].

5.2.2 Oxygen saturation (SaO2)

Arterial SaO2 is defined as the percentage of oxygenated hemoglobin (oxyhemo-globin) versus total hemoglobin (sum of oxyhemoglobin and deoxyhemoglobin). In the absence of hemoximetry capability, SaO2 is calculated using pH, PO2, and hemoglobin values.

5.2.3 Oxygen content

Oxygen content is defined as the total amount of oxygen in whole blood, including oxygen bound to hemoglobin and dissolved oxygen. Oxygen content is a combination of the amount of oxygen bound to hemoglobin and the amount of oxygen dissolved in the blood. Hemoglobin-bound oxygen is calculated by multi-plying the carrying capacity of one gram of hemoglobin (1.34 ml), with the amount of available hemoglobin (grams per deciliter) and oxygen saturation (SO2) [37].

$$O2\ Content = (1.34 \times Hemoglobin \times SO2) + (0.003 \times PO2) \tag{4}$$

5.3 Metabolites

Various metabolites such as glucose, lactate, creatinine, and bilirubin can be measured by blood gas analyzer using enzyme-based biosensors. These sensors exploit amperometric methods, which change the electrical conductivity of the solution following an oxidation-reduction reaction [38]. These metabolites indicate the accumulation or breakdown of chemical components in the body that indicate pulmonary status or disease condition.

5.4 Electrolytes

Analyzer can further measure the level of blood plasma electrolytes, such as sodium (Na^+), potassium (K^+) calcium (Ca^{++}) cations, and chloride anion (Cl^{--}), by ion-selective electrodes (ISE). These electrodes utilize a semi-permeable membrane for each ion, creating different concentrations and an electrical potential from which the concentration of the free ion is measured [39].

5.5 Other parameters

Analyzer can further calculate the additional parameters by combining the measured results and applied calculations to provide more information.

5.5.1 Bicarbonate (HCO3)

Blood gas analyzer calculates HCO3 concentration in arterial blood using measured values of pH and PCO2. Bicarbonate is a physiological buffer in body fluids that is produced from CO2 and H2O in the presence of carbonic anhydrase, and is part of a system that includes carbonic acid, carbonate, and carbon dioxide contributing to maintain pH balance. The calculation of the HCO3 value is based on the Henderson-Hasselbalch equation [40]. The range of normal values for HCO3 is 22–26 mEq/L.

5.5.2 Base excess/deficit

Analyzer can also calculate the relative excess (or deficit) of the base according to the measured pH and HCO3 values, which is a parameter used to assess the metabolic contribution in acid-base disorders. This parameter is defined as the titratable acid concentration required to titrate blood to pH 7.4 at 37°C, and 40 mmHg PCO2 [41]. Base excess is normally between −4 and + 2.

5.5.3 Anion gap

The anion gap is the difference between the measured cations and the measured anions. The most common use of the anion gap is to classify cases of metabolic acidosis. Specifically, classification into those with and those without unmeasured anions in plasma. In fact, the anion gap is a calculation that provides clinicians with the forethought to manage current problems associated with acid-base balance, fluids, and electrolytes.

The calculation is based on the measurement of specific cations, Na + and K+, and specific anions, Cl- and HCO3-, using the following equation:

$$\text{Anion gap} = \left(Na^+ + K^+\right) - \left(Cl^- + HCO3^-\right) \tag{5}$$

The anion gap equation can be further manipulated to reveal the presence of unmeasured cations and anions. The human body is electrically neutral, and thus, it does not have a true anion gap. Calculation of the anion gap is then useful to reveal changes in that balance. However, changes in albumin and bicarbonate concentrations require special attention. A normal anion gap is between 4 and 12 mmol/L, and majorly depends on serum concentrations of phosphate and albumin. An increased anion gap, or anion gap metabolic acidosis, is usually due to excess acid and/or base depletion. The decrease in the anion gap is mostly due to the decrease in albumin concentration because albumin is the primary unmeasured anion [42].

5.5.4 Osmolality and osmolar gap

Osmolality is the number of dissolved particles in a fluid. A blood osmolality test measures the amount of dissolved substances such as sodium, potassium, chloride, glucose, and urea in a blood sample. The most common application of serum osmolality is to detect poisoning or overdose induced by ingestion of toxins such as methanol (methyl alcohol), ethylene glycol, isopropyl alcohol, propylene glycol, acetone, and drugs such as salicylates (aspirin). As these toxins are osmotically active, the presence of the osmolar gap (osmotic gap) has been accepted as a screening test.

The osmolar gap is the difference between measured serum osmolality and calculated (estimated) osmolality results, which is estimated from the measurable osmotically active substances in the serum, including sodium, potassium, urea, glucose, and ethanol (alcohol).

$$\text{Calculated Osmolality} = \left(2x\left[\text{Sodium mmol}/L\right]\right) + \left[\text{urea mmol}/L\right] \\ \left[\text{glucose mmol}/L\right] + \left[\text{ethanol mmol}/L\right] \tag{6}$$

$$\text{Osmolar Gap} = \text{Measured Osmolality} - \text{Calculated Osmolality} \tag{7}$$

Normally, the osmolar gap is less than 10, and an osmolar gap above 10 can reflect the presence of abnormal substances (such as toxic alcohol) [43].

6. Sample collection and handling

Blood gas analysis can be performed on blood samples collected from several sites within the circulatory system, including arteries, veins, and capillaries. The specimen for arterial blood gas analysis is whole blood, obtained via arterial puncture or an indwelling arterial catheter. The dorsal pedal or femoral arteries are the predominant locations for arterial specimens; however, the coccyx and auricular arteries may also be utilized for sampling [44].

Specimens for venous blood gas analysis can be obtained from the jugular, saphenous, and cephalic veins. Central sites, such as venous catheters in the jugular vein, are generally preferred for sampling due to the fact that they provide a more comprehensive understanding of the patient's acid-base status. It is important to note that changes in local tissue perfusion can impact blood samples obtained from peripheral veins [45].

The selection of the sample collection location, whether artery or vein, should be determined by the diagnostic requirements during patient evaluation and the feasibility of sampling. The combination of venous blood gas analysis with pulse oximetry often provides sufficient data, making the challenges of arterial sampling and the additional stress it causes on the patient unjustified [31]. In the absence of an artery cannula or when repeated arterial punctures are to be avoided, arterialized capillary blood serves as an acceptable alternative to arterial blood, as capillary blood gases can reliably mimic their arterial analogues [46].

Arterial or venous samples should be collected anaerobically by sterile 1- to 3-mL syringes with lyophilized heparin anticoagulant. The anaerobic collection method refers to not exposing blood to atmospheric air. The PCO_2 of air is approximately 0.25 mm Hg, significantly lower than the PCO_2 in blood, which is around 40 mm Hg. Consequently, the CO_2 content and PCO_2 of blood exposed to air diminish, resulting in an increase in blood pH, which is dependent on PCO_2. The PO_2 of atmospheric air (155 mm Hg) exceeds arterial blood by approximately 60 mm Hg and is nearly 100 mm Hg higher in oxygen content. In contrast, blood with a PO_2 greater than 150 mm Hg, commonly observed in patients undergoing oxygen therapy, facilitates the release of oxygen [47, 48].

Small air bubbles may influence blood gas measurements. Blood can easily become exposed to air through the air inside the needle and the dead space of the syringe hub. The resulting bubble must be removed after drawing by holding the syringe tip up and emptying a small amount of blood, and the sample must be sealed to prevent air exposure. If the bubble is eliminated immediately, the mistake will be reduced [49]. Variations in syringe construction can cause significant differences in pre-analytical effects on the sample [50].

Lyophilized heparin anticoagulant is preferred over its liquid form because liquid heparin incorporates atmospheric PO_2 and PCO_2 values that dilute the sample. This effect is more significant when the syringe is not filled. Moreover, a higher ratio of liquid heparin to blood can have an increasing effect on the measured PCO_2 and the calculated parameters derived from it [51]. Evacuated lithium heparin sample tubes (vacuum tubes) utilized for plasma collection are undesirable due to the residual oxygen they contain, which compromises the accuracy of whole blood PO_2 readings [52].

Once obtained, the samples must be introduced for analysis within 15 minutes, otherwise, the samples should be placed on ice to slow the degradation of the gaseous components and analyzed as soon as possible to decrease the possibility of erroneous results. Before introducing the sample for analysis, it should be rewarmed to room temperature [53].

Since blood gas analyzers process whole blood, it is important to maintain complete homogeneity of the sample to ensure complete mixing and avoid sedimentation of red blood cells from the liquid plasma. Prior to gas analysis, mixing the sample by vigorously rotating the syringe between the palms must be done to create a homogeneous sample [54].

7. Quality control and calibration

Proper quality control (QC) and calibration are essential for the maintenance of blood gas analyzer, especially when decisions about critically ill patients are made based on the results obtained from this equipment. Calibration ensures accurate results and verifies that the analyzer is working properly. The following points will describe some tips to ensure consistent and accurate results based on the main parts of the blood gas analyzer.

7.1 Sample input

The syringes and glass or flexible capillary tubes of specimens are accepted by the sample input port. The machine pump typically draws 70–140 μl of blood into the sample holder for processing. At this stage, it is very important that air does not enter the sample path and has a good seal between the port and the sample. The most frequent reasons for air entry are a tear in the flexible port assembly, broken capillary glass, a worn o-ring, blood clots, or a hole in the flexible tubing. Most analyzer preventive maintenance (PM) kits provide all the components required to rebuild the assembly [36].

7.2 Calibration gas and reagent bank

Current analyzers have auto-calibration characteristics to ensure proper electrode response and accuracy, reducing the maintenance requirements for staff. They also incorporate solutions within sealed units, hence removing the necessity for gas cylinders and humidifiers. These solutions comprise standard reference materials with established concentrations of oxygen and carbon dioxide. The user can conduct 1-point or 2-point calibrations; 1-point calibration modifies the electrodes at either the high or low level, while 2-point calibration adjusts the electrodes at both levels. These calibrations may be scheduled for periodic execution or conducted prior to each measurement [31]. The manual calibration is a critical tool for the Biomedical equipment technicians (BMET) as special programs in the analyzer allowing the electronic analog and digital values of the electrodes to be viewed and utilized for electrode troubleshooting. The clinical laboratory further conducts external quality assurance validations to verify the accuracy of the blood gas system, which is usually considered as last step after maintenance or repair [36].

7.3 Washing and rinsing bank

This subset keeps clear and clean fluid paths. Washing is performed after each sample to avoid cross-contamination between experiments. As an additional feature, in most analyzer wash processes, air slugs are intentionally introduced into the sample port, which creates turbulence and a scraping action on the fluid tube walls to improve the wash performance. When troubleshooting this part, attention should be paid to the air/fluid pattern and noise of this cycle. With practice, it is possible to determine whether the fluid paths indicate air leaks or occlusions [36].

Peripheral venous blood gas analysis versus arterial blood gas analysis for the diagnosis Troubleshooting Common Issues:

Arterial and venous samples can be used for blood gas analysis. An arterial blood gas (ABG) expressly examines blood drawn from an artery. An ABG test requires a small volume of blood to be taken from the radial artery, however, arterial samples can also be obtained from the femoral artery or from an arterial catheter [55]. Although an arterial sample requires more advanced technical skills to obtain, it is less likely to result in inaccuracies due to poor perfusion compared to a venous sample [31]. ABG analysis evaluates the PaO2 and PaCO2 of the patient's blood [56].

The evaluation of PaO2 offers data on oxygenation status, and PaCO2 provides data on ventilation status (chronic or acute respiratory failure) [47].

Venous samples are most easily obtained by either direct venipuncture or an intra-venous catheter. They can be utilized to assess metabolic and electrolyte imbalances, offering insights into the patient's breathing condition; nevertheless, these samples are ineffective for evaluating oxygenation status [57]. The gas values of venous blood can be affected by changes in metabolism and peripheral circulation, and they can reflect the metabolic activity of tissues distal to the sample collection site. Thus, central venous samples are preferred over peripheral venous samples, however, more data can be obtained from peripheral venous blood gas in well-perfused patients [31].

Moreover, it is important to know the type of sample as venous and arterial samples have differences in measured blood gas values. These differences are more pronounced for PO2 because PO2 is the only clinical reason to obtain arterial collections [58]. After capillary O2 release, PO2 is typically approximately 60 mmHg lower in venous blood, whereas, venous PCO2 is often nearly 5 mmHg higher than arterial PCO2. The pH is usually 0.02 to 0.05 pH units higher in the arterial samples [59].

8. Advancements in sampling technology

ABG testing is essential in critical care and respiratory medicine for assessing a patient's oxygenation, ventilation, and acid-base status. Traditionally, ABG analysis required cumbersome procedures and waiting times, posing risks in urgent care scenarios. However, recent technological advancements have revolutionized this process, offering rapid, accurate, and less invasive testing methods [60]. Innovations in blood gas and electrolyte analyzers are transforming patient care through the implementation of non-invasive sampling methods and enhanced sensor technology. These advancements have multiple advantages, including improved accuracy and sensitivity in measurements, greater patient comfort, and reduced problems. Non-invasive sampling obviates the necessity for intrusive treatments, enhancing comfort during monitoring and facilitating frequent assessments.

Advancements in blood gas analysis have focused on improving sampling tech-nologies, particularly through the exploration of VBGs as alternatives to traditional ABGs. This shift addresses the challenges associated with arterial sampling, such as the difficulty of obtaining arterial blood due to patient movement or poor peripheral circulation.

VBGs can be collected from peripheral veins or central venous catheters, making them more accessible than arterial samples, especially in emergency and intensive care settings. Also, the risk of complications such as hemorrhage and arterial puncture pain is significantly lower with venous sampling. This makes VBGs a safer option for patients, particularly those requiring frequent blood gas assessments [61]. In addition, studies have shown that VBGs can provide comparable insights into systemic carbon dioxide and pH levels. For instance, research indicates that venous pH can effectively replace arterial pH in initial emergency assessments, particularly in patients with conditions like diabetic ketoacidosis [62].

Recent advancements include the development of automated real-time analysis systems for blood gas interpretation. These POCT devices improve the speed and accuracy of blood gas analysis, allowing for immediate clinical decision-making. They reduce turnaround times and minimize errors associated with traditional laboratory processes.

One of the significant advancements in ABG testing is the development of portable point-of-care devices. These compact, handheld units allow for bedside testing, reducing the time from sample collection to result interpretation. POC devices are equipped with user-friendly interfaces and require smaller blood volumes, which is particularly beneficial in pediatrics and for patients with limited vascular access [63]. On the other hand, emerging research is also exploring non-invasive methods, such as saliva sampling, to evaluate blood gas parameters like PaO2, PaCO2, pH, and HCO3. This method aims to provide a safer alternative to ABG sampling, especially in traumatic patients under mechanical ventilation. Preliminary studies suggest that salivary gas values correlate well with traditional ABG results, potentially expanding the utility of non-invasive testing in clinical practice [61]. As research continues, the integration of non-invasive methods like saliva sampling may further revolutionize how clinicians assess respiratory and metabolic statuses. Additionally, modern sensor technology improves reliability and accurately identifies even slight variations in concentration. This connection enhances patient care and facilitates real-time, continuous monitoring for individualized management. Consequently, it offers a favorable market environment, enhancing efficiency and healthcare results. Furthermore, modern ABG analyzers are designed to integrate seamlessly with Electronic Health Records (EHRs), enabling automatic data entry and reducing manual errors. This integration ensures that healthcare providers have immediate access to ABG results within a patient's comprehensive medical history, facilitating quicker and more informed clinical decisions [63–65].

Advancements in sampling technology have led to the development of various non-invasive methods to assess arterial blood gas tensions and pH, providing more convenient and patient-friendly alternatives to direct arterial catheterization. One potential substitute for arterial sampling is arterialized capillary blood, which may closely reflect arterial blood. By promoting vasodilation through topical vasodilatory substances or warming the sampling area, the differences between arterial and arterialized capillary blood may be reduced, making capillary sampling an attractive, less invasive option. This approach has been suggested for use in physiological exercise testing and in clinical settings for patients with respiratory disorders, as well as for endurance athletes to assess gas exchange abnormalities [66]. Despite the potential benefits of arterialized capillary blood sampling, there have been conflicting views on its accuracy compared to arterial blood. Some studies have shown agreement between arterialized samples and arterial blood at rest in both adults and children, while others have not demonstrated such agreement. Moreover, there has been an ongoing debate over the accuracy, precision, and usefulness of fingertip and earlobe capillary blood sampling in comparison to arterial blood sampling. As a result, a comprehensive understanding of the validity and reliability of arterialized capillary blood sampling is essential for its widespread adoption as an alternative to arterial blood sampling [66, 67]. In order to address these uncertainties, a meta-analysis was assumed to systematically review original research studies comparing arterial blood samples with arterialized capillary samples. The results of the meta-analysis indicated that arterialized capillary blood sampled from the earlobe was more accurate in reflecting arterial PO2 and PCO2 compared to blood sampled from the fingertip. This finding suggests that, in certain circumstances and conditions, arterialized capillary blood from the earlobe could provide a reliable substitute for arterial sampling. The study also identified the critical thresholds at which the mean differences between arterial and capillary samples are not significant, further indicating the contexts in which capillary sampling may provide accurate estimations of arterial values. Additionally, the meta-analysis revealed that the accuracy of capillary blood sampling is dependent on the arterial values, with the accuracy of a capillary sample to reflect arterial PO2 improving in hypoxic conditions [67]. Overall, the meta-analysis provided compelling evidence supporting the use of arterialized capillary blood sampled from the earlobe as a potential alternative to arterial blood sampling, particularly for assessing PO2 and PCO2. The findings offer valuable insights into the accuracy and reliability of capillary blood sampling technology, paving the way for its potential integration into various clinical applications. The advancements in sampling technology have played a crucial role in improving the accuracy and precision of point-of-care blood gas testing [68].

Overall, this advancement in sampling technology represents a significant improvement in the quality management of POC blood gas testing, providing real-time error detection and automatic correction of errors. It addresses the need for constant vigilance and safeguards against reporting erroneous results, ultimately enhancing the accuracy and reliability of POC testing.

9. Digital solutions and robotics in blood gas and electrolyte analyzer

The implementation of digital technology and robots in blood gas and electrolyte analyzers has transformed the methodology by which healthcare practitioners diagnose and monitor patient situations. These modern technologies have markedly enhanced the efficiency, precision, and simplicity of performing blood gas and electrolyte tests, thereby benefiting both patients and medical personnel. Digital technologies have expedited and automated data gathering and processing, minimizing human errors and improving the turnaround time for test findings. The advanced algorithms and machine learning capabilities of these analyzers facilitate the interpretation of complex data, resulting in faster and more accurate diagnoses than previously possible.

In 2020, Roche v-TAC introduced an advanced digital diagnostics solution enabling clinicians to obtain arterial blood gas measurements from patients requiring blood gas analysis. This approach is a simpler, less painful, and minimally invasive venous operation, offering a more comfortable experience for patients. Roche v-TAC is fully connected with Roche's cobas b 123 POC and cobas b 221 systems via the Roche cobas infinite POC solution. This uninterrupted communication ensures swift and accurate data transmission and reporting. It enhances the diagnostic process and improves patient care. The introduction of Roche v-TAC represents a significant advancement in blood gas analysis, offering a more patient-focused and accessible approach to obtaining critical diagnostic information [69, 70].

The implementation of digital technology and robotic process automation has become increasingly common in contemporary healthcare systems. These technologies possess the capacity to transform multiple facets of healthcare delivery, encompassing the optimization of administrative functions, the enhancement of patient care, and the augmentation of operational efficiency. Digital health solutions comprise many tools and services, such as telemedicine, electronic health records, patient portals, mobile health applications, and wearable devices. In clinical laboratories, automation and robotics facilitate high-throughput sample processing, minimizing human error and improving workflow efficiency [68].

In addition, the arterial blood gas algorithm introduces a digital diagnostics solution that offers real-time interpretation of preliminary data on safety features, oxygenation measurements, acid-base disturbances, and renal profile evaluations. This introduction aims to address the challenges associated with numerically reported test results from point-of-care arterial blood gas measurements, making rapid interpretation difficult or open to interpretation. The arterial blood gas algorithm software presents a new way to improve clinical outcomes by providing clinicians with automated analysis and interpretation of arterial blood gases, potentially reducing human errors and promptly identifying life-threatening situations. Additionally, the software can be integrated into medical devices or interfaces for seamless communication and integration of results with hospital information systems and other devices. The study focused on clinically validating the arterial blood gas algorithm against senior experienced clinicians for acid-base interpretation in a clinical context, demonstrating its potential as a reliable and clinically useful tool for POCT [27].

In this same subject and direction, the ongoing digital revolution in healthcare has introduced cutting-edge digital solutions and robotics to revolutionize the interpretation of blood gas tests. These contemporary technologies integrate artificial intelligence-based systems that have the potential to streamline and enhance the decision-making process in healthcare centers. By leveraging digital solutions and robotics, the interpretation of complex blood gas tests can become more efficient and accurate, ultimately contributing to improved patient care and outcomes. The integration of these technologies paves the way for the development of registries and artificial intelligence-based systems, which can further augment the capacity of healthcare professionals to make informed and timely decisions based on blood gas analysis data [64]. As a result, the introduction of digital solutions and robotics marks a significant advancement for the healthcare industry, promising to enhance the interpretation of blood gas tests and overall patient care [64].

10. Quality assurance and method verification in blood gas analysis

Quality assurance and method verification are critical components of laboratory practice, ensuring the accuracy and reliability of diagnostic test results, particularly in critical areas such as blood gas analysis. Quality assurance encompasses the systematic measures and processes put in place to maintain and improve the quality of laboratory testing, ensuring that the results generated are both accurate and consistent. One essential aspect of quality assurance in laboratory testing is the establishment and monitoring of quality control procedures, which includes the verification of assay performance and compliance with regulatory standards [71, 72].

11. Method verification

Method verification involves the assessment and confirmation of the performance characteristics of an assay or analytical method. It ensures that the method used in the laboratory is suitable for its intended purpose and provides reliable results. In the context of blood gas analysis, method verification would involve assessing parameters such as accuracy, precision, analytical sensitivity, and specificity of the blood gas analyzer [72].

12. Quality control in blood gas analysis

QC is an essential component of a laboratory's quality plan, and ensuring the accuracy and precision of blood gas analyzers is crucial for patient care. Assayed QC materials, which come with manufacturer-provided mean values and ranges, are commonly used for QC testing in blood gas analysis. However, it is important for laboratories to verify the accuracy of these manufacturer-provided QC mean values and ranges to ensure that they are appropriate for their specific blood gas analyzer. The verification of tested QC ranges is a requirement of the Clinical Laboratory Improvement Amendments (CLIA) and is essential for conforming to quality assurance and patient safety standards. Furthermore, the American Association for Respiratory Care (AARC) Clinical Practice Guideline emphasizes the necessity of validating and modifying QC mean values and ranges to align with the analyzer's performance [71, 72].

13. Advances in quality control technology

QC testing is an essential element of point-of-care blood gas analysis to ensure accurate and exact outcomes. The GEM Premier 5000, equipped with next-generation Intelligent Quality Management 2 (iQM2), was assessed for its efficacy in monitoring more than 84,000 patient samples across four locations. The researchers evaluated the efficacy of continuous iQM2 testing compared to intermittent liquid QC, focusing on method precision, sigma, error detection probability, false rejection probability, and average error detection time. The study's findings revealed that the superior performance of the GEM Premier 5000 with iQM2, exhibiting above six sigma precision for all analytes and expedited error detection times, especially when contrasted with intermittent liquid QC methods [68, 71].

A previous study aimed to assess the efficacy of Intelligent Quality Management 2 (iQM2) on the GEM Premier 5000 for error identification and automatic elimination of errors, comprising those resulting from both pre-analytical and analytical testing phases. Additionally, the previous studies compared the error-detection capabilities of continuous iQM2 testing versus intermittent QC testing. Generation Intelligent Quality Management 2 (iQM2) refers to the next-generation quality management system used in the evaluation of the GEM Premier 5000 point-of-care blood gas testing system. It offers continuous monitoring and rapid error detection to ensure high accuracy and precision in test results. This technology utilizes continuous quality checks throughout the testing process to ensure the accuracy of sample measurement, focusing on hardware, software, and analytical functionality. It combines innovative pattern-recognition algorithms and IntraSpectTM technology, which detects sensor patterns related to errors during the sample measurement process. This includes identifying transient errors such as micro-clots, micro-bubbles, and interferences that could affect the analytical performance of the analyzer. These types of errors can go undetected with traditional liquid-based quality control (QC) processes, thereby potentially leading to erroneous results [68, 73].

iQM2 technology was able to identify potential pre-analytical errors, including both systemic and transient errors at the point of care. It demonstrated precision and efficiency in detecting errors that may negatively impact patient care. The study examined the method sigma and average detection time (ADT) for an error to compare the performance of continuous iQM2 with intermittent liquid QC, either manual or automated. Continuous iQM2 exhibited faster error detection times, with an average detection time of approximately 2 minutes, compared to intermittent liquid QC, which varied from hours to days. Additionally, iQM2 process control solutions (PCS) precision was found to be similar to or better than manual or automated internal QC for all analytes, with greater than six sigma precision. The findings demonstrate that the GEM Premier 5000 with iQM2 offers excellent performance, including greater than six sigma precision for all analytes and faster error detection times. The technology was able to detect errors in approximately 1.4% of samples, providing an additional safeguard against reporting erroneous results [68, 74].

Moreover, the results indicated that this continuous quality monitoring procedure exhibited markedly quicker mistake detection times relative to intermittent QC methods, with average detection times of approximately 2 minutes for iQM2, in contrast to hours or even days for intermittent QC. The iQM2 technology not only identified problems but also promptly alerted the operator and commenced corrective measures to rectify sample-specific faults within minutes. This prompt reaction reduced the effect on system availability, resulting in merely 0.186% or 43 minutes of downtime for the average lifespan of the GEM PAK. These advantages decrease risks at various stages of testing that are not readily identifiable with sporadic liquid quality control (human or automated). This is crucial for ensuring the precision and dependability of point-of-care blood gas analysis [68].

14. Clinical implications of blood gas analysis

Quality assurance and method verification in blood gas analysis are critical for accurate diagnosis and treatment in clinical settings. Ensuring the reliability of blood gas measurements directly impacts patient care, particularly in emergency and intensive care environments. Blood gas QC is essential, requiring laboratories to verify manufacturer-provided QC ranges against their own measurements. A study found that 71% of comparisons showed less than 1% difference, yet none of the manufacturer ranges were clinically acceptable [72]. Blood gas analysis has evolved significantly, with modern analyzers capable of rapid, multi-parameter testing, crucial for timely diagnosis in critical care [75]. POCT has been shown to enhance diagnostic accuracy and treatment quality in pre-hospital settings, allowing for immediate assessment of respiratory and acid-base disorders [76, 77]. Differences between POCT and central laboratory results can lead to misdiagnosis, particularly for parameters like pO2, highlighting the importance of timely analysis [78]. The strong ion approach provides a more nuanced understanding of acid-base disturbances, aiding in targeted treatment strategies [79]. While advancements in blood gas analysis have improved diagnostic capabilities, the potential for discrepancies between testing methods necessitates careful interpretation and verification to ensure optimal patient outcomes.

Taken together, quality assurance is critical in blood gas analysis to ensure accurate and reliable results that guide patient diagnosis and treatment. Key aspects of quality assurance include:

Verification of Assayed QC Ranges: Laboratories must verify manufacturer-provided QC mean values and ranges for blood gas analyzers, even when using assayed QC materials. This is a requirement under the Clinical Laboratory Improvement Amendment (CLIA). The laboratory should calculate its own mean and 2 SD ranges from repetitive testing and adjust QC ranges to match the analyzer's performance. Studies have shown that manufacturer-provided ranges are often much wider than the actual 2 SD ranges, ranging from 2.4 to 75 SD from the measured mean. Using unverified ranges could allow analyzer malfunctions to go undetected, potentially impacting patient care [72, 80].

Calibration Verification: Calibration verification should be performed in various situations, including when a complete change of reagents is introduced, after major preventive maintenance or critical part replacements, if quality control results indicate a problem, after an environmental change or instrument relocation, when an instrument is replaced, or if QC materials show an unusual trend or are outside acceptable limits. The laboratory must establish its own QC ranges with valid statistical measurements for each test [80, 81].

Continuous Quality Monitoring: Real-time error detection systems like Intelligent Quality Management (iQM) can provide continuous monitoring of blood gas analyzers. Studies show that iQM detects errors in about 1.4% of samples and provides faster error detection times compared to intermittent liquid QC. This addresses risks in different phases of testing that may be missed by periodic QC alone [68].

In summary, verifying QC ranges, performing calibration verification, and implementing continuous quality monitoring are essential to ensure the accuracy and reliability of blood gas analysis. This promotes patient safety by providing high-quality data to guide diagnosis and treatment decisions. Quality assurance and method verification are fundamental principles in laboratory medicine, playing a pivotal role in safeguarding the accuracy of diagnostic test results. In the context of blood gas analysis, these processes are essential for ensuring the reliability and validity of blood gas measurements, ultimately contributing to patient safety and effective clinical decision-making.

15. Conclusion

Blood gas analysis is a valuable component in the diagnostic evaluation of the critically ill patient. Blood gas analysis provides data on oxygenation, ventilation, and acid-base status that may be difficult to perceive in clinical examination findings or routine monitoring devices. A blood gas analysis also provides testing of a number of values, such as electrolytes, blood glucose, and hemoglobin. Interpretation is performed in a systematic manner to detect the primary disorder, secondary disorders, and thus differential diagnoses that can contribute to the patient's clinical condition.

Considering the various models of blood gas analyzers and their different measurement capabilities, it is recommended to spend time researching and finding the ideal device for a specific procedure. After purchase, staff training in sample collection, sample handling, maintenance of instruments, and quality control is important for the efficiency and accuracy of the results, which can also raise the level of care in practice.

Authors' contributions

Conceptualization: MM. Data curation: AEN and MA. Writing-original draft: MM, MT, AEN, and MA. Writing-review and editing: MT, MM. Analysis and/or interpretation of data: MM and MT. All authors read and approved the final manuscript.

Competing interests

The authors declare that they have no competing interests.

Abbreviations

ABG	arterial blood gas
AARC	American Association for Respiratory Care
BMET	Biomedical equipment technicians
CLIA	clinical laboratory improvement amendment
COPD	chronic obstructive pulmonary disease
DKA	diabetic ketoacidosis
EHRs	electronic health records
EPOC	enterprise point-of-care
iQM	intelligent quality management
ICU	intensive care units
POCT	point-of-care testing
QC	quality control
VBGs	venous blood gases

Author details

Marjan Taherian[1], Mojtaba Ahmadlou[2], Asieh Emami Nejad[3]* and Mostafa Manian[4,5]*

1 Cellular and Molecular Research Center, Iran University of Medical Sciences, Tehran, Iran

2 Department of Biostatistics, School of Medicine, Arak University of Medical Sciences, Arak, Iran

3 Department of Biology, Payame Noor University (PNU), Tehran, Iran

4 Department of Medical Laboratory Science, Faculty of Medical Science Kermanshah Branch, Islamic Azad University, Kermanshah, Iran

5 Isfahan Neurosciences Research Center, Alzahra Research Institute, Isfahan University of Medical Sciences, Isfahan, Iran

*Address all correspondence to: emami_asieh@yahoo.com
and mostafamanian@gmail.com

IntechOpen

References

[1] Gross R, Peruzzi W. Chapter 14 - Arterial blood gas measurements. In: Parrillo JE, Dellinger RP, editors. Critical Care Medicine. 3rd ed. Philadelphia: Mosby; 2008. pp. 233-253

[2] Venkatesh B. Chapter 42 - In-line blood gas monitoring. In: Papadakos PJ, Lachmann B, Visser-Isles L, editors. Mechanical Ventilation. Philadelphia: W.B. Saunders; 2008. pp. 487-499

[3] Gattinoni L, Pesenti A, Matthay M. Understanding blood gas analysis. Intensive Care Medicine. 2018;**44**(1):91-93

[4] Elmeshreghi TN et al. Comparison of enterprise point-of-care and Nova biomedical critical care Xpress analyzers for determination of arterial pH, blood gas, and electrolyte values in canine and equine blood. Veterinary Clinical Pathology. 2018;**47**(3):415-424

[5] Agarwal S et al. Evaluation of the analytical performance of the modified enterprise point-of-care blood gas and electrolyte analyzer in a pediatric hospital. Point of Care. 2014;**13**(4):132-136

[6] Gutierres SL, Welty TE. Point-of-care testing: An introduction. Annals of Pharmacotherapy. 2004;**38**(1):119-125

[7] Tinkey P et al. Use of the i-STAT portable clinical analyzer in mice. Lab Animal. 2006;**35**(2):45-50

[8] Silverman S, Birks E. Evaluation of the i-STAT hand-held chemical analyser during treadmill and endurance exercise. Equine Veterinary Journal. 2002;**34**(S34):551-554

[9] Myers GJ, Browne J. Point of care hematocrit and hemoglobin in cardiac surgery: A review. Perfusion. 2007;**22**(3):179-183

[10] Kapoor D, Srivastava M, Singh P. Point of care blood gases with electrolytes and lactates in adult emergencies. International Journal of Critical Illness and Injury Science. 2014;**4**(3):216-222

[11] Cox CJ. Acute care testing: Blood gases and electrolytes at the point of care. Clinics in Laboratory Medicine. 2001;**21**(2):321-336

[12] Nichols JH et al. Executive summary. The National Academy of Clinical Biochemistry Laboratory medicine practice guideline: Evidence-based practice for point-of-care testing. Clinica Chimica Acta. 2007;**379**(1-2):14-28; discussion 29-30

[13] Chance JJ et al. Multiple site analytical evaluation of a portable blood gas/electrolyte analyzer for point of care testing. Critical Care Medicine. 2000;**28**(6):2081-2085

[14] Flegar-Mestrić Z, Perkov S. Comparability of point-of-care whole-blood electrolyte and substrate testing using a Stat profile critical care Xpress analyzer and standard laboratory methods. Clinical Chemistry and Laboratory Medicine. 2006;**44**(7):898-903

[15] Jain A, Subhan I, Joshi M. Comparison of the point-of-care blood gas analyzer versus the laboratory auto-analyzer for the measurement of electrolytes. International Journal of Emergency Medicine. 2009;**2**(2):117-120

[16] Konstantinov NK et al. Respiratory failure in diabetic ketoacidosis. World Journal of Diabetes. 2015;**6**(8):1009-1023

[17] Jung W et al. Point-of-care testing (POCT) diagnostic systems using microfluidic lab-on-a-chip technologies. Microelectronic Engineering. 2015;**132**: 46-57

[18] Abuzinadah AR, Almalki AK, Almuteeri RZ, Althalabi RH, Sahli HA, Hayash FA, et al. Utility of initial arterial blood gas in neuromuscular versus non-neuromuscular acute respiratory failure in intensive care unit patients. Journal of Clinical Medicine. 2022;**11**(16):4926. DOI: 10.3390/jcm11164926

[19] Ozsancak Ugurlu A, Habesoglu MA. Epidemiology of NIV for acute respiratory failure in COPD patients: Results from the international surveys vs. the "real world". COPD. 2017;**14**(4):429-438

[20] Streets AM, Huang Y. Chip in a lab: Microfluidics for next generation life science research. Biomicrofluidics. Jan 2013;**7**(1):11302. DOI: 10.1063/1.4789751. Epub 2013 Jan 31

[21] Kempker JA et al. The epidemiology of respiratory failure in the United States 2002-2017: A serial cross-sectional study. Critical Care Explorations. 2020;**2**(6):e0128

[22] Chuang ML, Hsieh BY, Lin IF. Prediction and types of dead-space fraction during exercise in male chronic obstructive pulmonary disease patients. Medicine (Baltimore). 2022;**101**(6):e28800

[23] Kraut JA, Kurtz I. Toxic alcohol ingestions: Clinical features, diagnosis, and management. Clinical Journal of the American Society of Nephrology. 2008;**3**(1):208-225

[24] Kabli AO et al. Outcome of methanol toxicity outbreak In Saudi Arabia: Case series study. Cureus. 2023;**15**(6):e41108

[25] Sista R et al. Development of a digital microfluidic platform for point of care testing. Lab on a Chip. 2008;**8**(12):2091-2104

[26] Streets AM, Huang Y. Microfluidics for biological measurements with single-molecule resolution. Current Opinion in Biotechnology. 2014;**25**:69-77

[27] Rodríguez-Villar S et al. Automatic real-time analysis and interpretation of arterial blood gas sample for point-of-care testing: Clinical validation. PLoS One. 2021;**16**(3):e0248264

[28] Haskins S. An Overview of Acid-Base Physiology. 1977

[29] Eknoyan G. Acid–base homeostasis: A historical inquiry of its origins and conceptual evolution. Nephrology Dialysis Transplantation. 2022;**37**(10):1816-1823

[30] Adams A, Morgan-Hughes J, Sykes M. pH and blood—Gas analysis: Methods of measurement and sources of error using electrode systems part 1. Anaesthesia. 1967;**22**(4):575-597

[31] Gonzalez AL, Waddell LS. Blood gas analyzers. Topics in Companion Animal Medicine. 2016;**31**(1):27-34

[32] DiBartola SP. Introduction to acid-base disorders. In: Fluid, Electrolyte, and Acid-Base Disorders in Small Animal Practice. 2012. pp. 231-252

[33] Rose BD, Post T. Clinical Physiology of Acid-Base and Electrolyte Disorders. McGraw Hill LLC; 2001

[34] Severinghaus JW, Bradley AF. Electrodes for blood pO2 and pCO2 determination. Journal of Applied Physiology. 1958;**13**(3):515-520

[35] Reynafarje B, Costa LE, Lehninger AL. O2 solubility in aqueous

media determined by a kinetic method. Analytical Biochemistry. 1985;**145**(2):406-418

[36] Stiles DA. Blood gas analyzers. Biomedical Instrumentation and Technology. 2007;**41**(5):377-378

[37] Rieser TM. Arterial and venous blood gas analyses. Topics in Companion Animal Medicine. 2013;**28**(3):86-90

[38] D'Orazio P. Biosensors in clinical chemistry. Clinica Chimica Acta. 2003;**334**(1-2):41-69

[39] Albert V et al. Agreement of two different laboratory methods used to measure electrolytes. Journal of Laboratory Physicians. 2011;**3**(02):104-109

[40] Constable PD. Clinical assessment of acid-base status: Comparison of the Henderson-Hasselbalch and strong ion approaches. Veterinary Clinical Pathology. 2000;**29**(4):115-128

[41] Camacho M et al. Acid-base and plasma biochemical changes using crystalloid fluids in stranded juvenile loggerhead sea turtles (Caretta caretta). PLoS One. 2015;**10**(7):e0132217

[42] Pandey DG, Sharma S. Biochemistry, anion gap. 2023 Jul 10. In: StatPearls [Internet]. Treasure Island (FL): StatPearls Publishing; 2024

[43] Purssell RA, Lynd LD, Koga Y. The use of the osmole gap as a screening test for the presence of exogenous substances. Toxicological Reviews. 2004;**23**(3):189-202

[44] Todorović J, Nešovic-Ostojić J, Milovanović A, Brkić P, Ille M, Čemerikić D. The assessment of acid-base analysis: Comparison of the "traditional" and the "modern"

approaches. Medicinski Glasnik: Official Publication of the Medical Association of Zenica-Doboj Canton, Bosnia and Herzegovina. 2015;**12**(1):7-18

[45] Treger R et al. Agreement between central venous and arterial blood gas measurements in the intensive care unit. Clinical Journal of the American Society of Nephrology. 2010;**5**(3):390-394

[46] Kirubakaran C, Gnananayagam JE, Sundaravalli EK. Comparison of blood gas values in arterial and venous blood. Indian Journal of Pediatrics. 2003;**70**(10):781-785

[47] Castro D, Patil SM, Zubair M, Keenaghan M. Arterial blood gas. In: StatPearls [Internet]. Treasure Island (FL): StatPearls Publishing; 2024

[48] Knowles TP et al. Effects of syringe material, sample storage time, and temperature on blood gases and oxygen saturation in arterialized human blood samples. Respiratory Care. 2006;**51**(7):732-736

[49] Çuhadar S et al. Detection of preanalytical errors in arterial blood gas analysis. Biochemia Medica (Zagreb). 2022;**32**(2):020708

[50] Sood P, Paul G, Puri S. Interpretation of arterial blood gas. Indian Journal of Critical Care Medicine. 2010;**14**(2):57-64

[51] Jiang HX. The effect of dilution and heparin on the blood gas analysis. Zhonghua Jie He He Hu Xi Za Zhi. 1992;**15**(4):225-227 255-6

[52] Higgins C. The use of heparin in preparing samples for blood-gas analysis. MLO: Medical Laboratory Observer. 2007;**39**(10):16-18, 20; quiz 22-3

[53] Dev SP, Hillmer MD, Ferri M. Videos in clinical medicine. Arterial puncture

for blood gas analysis. The New England Journal of Medicine. 2011;**364**(5):e7

[54] Lima-Oliveira G et al. Different manufacturers of syringes: A new source of variability in blood gas, acid-base balance and related laboratory test? Clinical Biochemistry. 2012;**45**(9):683-687

[55] Lian JX. Interpreting and using the arterial blood gas analysis. Nursing 2020 Critical Care. 2010;**5**(3):26-36

[56] Ziegenfuß T, Zander R. Understanding blood gas analysis. Intensive Care Medicine. 2019;**45**(11):1684-1685. DOI: 10.1007/s00134-019-05688-w. Epub 2019 Aug 7

[57] Haskins SC. Chapter 25 - Interpretation of blood gas measurements. In: King LG, editor. Textbook of Respiratory Disease in Dogs and Cats. Saint Louis: W.B. Saunders; 2004. pp. 181-193

[58] Malatesha G et al. Comparison of arterial and venous pH, bicarbonate, PCO2 and PO2 in initial emergency department assessment. Emergency Medicine Journal. 2007;**24**(8):569-571

[59] Magnet FS et al. Capillary PO(2) does not adequately reflect arterial PO(2) in hypoxemic COPD patients. International Journal of Chronic Obstructive Pulmonary Disease. 2017;**12**:2647-2653

[60] Boulain T et al. Predicting arterial blood gas and lactate from central venous blood analysis in critically ill patients: A multicentre, prospective, diagnostic accuracy study. British Journal of Anaesthesia. 2016;**117**(3):341-349

[61] Hamid HS, Babak A, Leyla R, Kahrizsangi MS, Nazemroaya B. The use of saliva sample evaluating PaO$_2$, PaCO$_2$, pH, and HCO$_3$ values in traumatic

patients under mechanical ventilation, as a non-invasive approach than the arterial blood gas sampling. Archives of Anesthesiology and Critical Care [Internet]. 2022;**8**(4):274-279. Available from: https://sid.ir/paper/1010980/en

[62] Byrne AL et al. Peripheral venous blood gas analysis versus arterial blood gas analysis for the diagnosis of respiratory failure and metabolic disturbance in adults. Cochrane Database of Systematic Reviews. 2013;**2013**(11):CD010841. DOI: 10.1002/14651858.CD010841. eCollection 2013 Nov

[63] Honarmand A, Safavi M. Prediction of arterial blood gas values from arterialized earlobe blood gas values in patients treated with mechanical ventilation. Indian Journal of Critical Care Medicine. 2008;**12**(3):96-101

[64] Zare S et al. Identification of data elements for blood gas analysis dataset: A base for developing registries and artificial intelligence-based systems. BMC Health Services Research. 2022;**22**(1):317

[65] Ambinder EP. Electronic health records. Journal of Oncology Practice/American Society of Clinical Oncology. 2005;**1**(2):57-63

[66] Hoffman MSF et al. Minimally invasive capillary blood sampling methods. Expert Review of Medical Devices. 2023;**20**(1):5-16

[67] Zavorsky GS et al. Arterial versus capillary blood gases: A meta-analysis. Respiratory Physiology and Neurobiology. 2007;**155**(3):268-279

[68] Nichols JH et al. Clinical validation of a novel quality management system for blood gas, electrolytes, metabolites, and CO-oximetry. Journal

of Applied Laboratory Medicine. 2021;**6**(6):1396-1408

[69] Yang Z, Zhou DMJCB. Cardiac markers and their point-of-care testing for diagnosis of acute myocardial infarction. 2006;**39**(8):771-780

[70] Althobiani M et al. S120 adherence and quality of home-based spirometry in patients with ILD using a digital health platform during a 6-month period: Data from the RALPMH study. 2022;**77**(Suppl 1):A74-A75

[71] Toffaletti JG. Upping the game on validating automatic quality management systems for blood gas and critical care test analyzers. Journal of Applied Laboratory Medicine. 2021;**6**(6):1393-1395

[72] Haynes JM, Fishwick RG. Verification of assayed blood gas quality control ranges. Respiratory Care. 2022;**67**(4):428-432

[73] Westgard JO, Cervera J. Intelligent quality management 2 with IntraSpect™ technology for quality control of GEM® premier™ 5000 blood gas analyzers- a novel application of the patient sample as its own control. Practical Laboratory Medicine. 2022;**30**:e00273

[74] van Rossum HH. Technical quality assurance and quality control for medical laboratories: A review and proposal of a new concept to obtain integrated and validated QA/QC plans. Critical Reviews in Clinical Laboratory Sciences. 2022;**59**(8):586-600

[75] Chen C et al. Applications of multi-omics analysis in human diseases. 2023;**4**(4):e315

[76] Chan JTN et al. Point-of-care testing in private pharmacy and drug retail settings: A narrative review. BMC Infectious Diseases. 2023;**23**(1):551

[77] Gao Q, Li S. Intelligent point of care testing for medicine diagnosis. 2024;**2**(1):e20230031

[78] Krzych L et al. Be cautious during the interpretation of arterial blood gas analysis performed outside the intensive care unit. Acta Biochimica Polonica. 2020;**67**(3):353-358

[79] Shreewastav RK et al. Study of Acid-Base disorders and biochemical findings of patients in a tertiary care hospital: A descriptive cross-sectional study. JNMA; Journal of the Nepal Medical Association. 2019;**57**(220):432-436

[80] Nichols JH. Quality in point-of-care testing. Expert Review of Molecular Diagnostics. 2003;**3**(5):563-572

[81] Plebani M. Does POCT reduce the risk of error in laboratory testing? Clinica Chimica Acta. 2009;**404**(1):59-64

Chapter 3

Blood Gas Monitoring in Anesthesia Applications

Semin Turhan

Abstract

This chapter provides a comprehensive overview of blood gas monitoring in anesthesia, focusing on various methods such as arterial blood gas (ABG) analysis, venous blood gas (VBG) analysis, and non-invasive monitoring techniques. The chapter discusses the importance of monitoring parameters like pH, PaCO$_2$, and PaO$_2$ during anesthesia to maintain respiratory and metabolic stability, and it highlights the differences between arterial and venous blood gases in clinical practice. Innovations in blood gas monitoring technologies, including transcutaneous monitoring, capnography, and artificial intelligence (AI)-supported digital systems, are explored, with emphasis on their impact on real-time decision-making and patient safety. The future role of artificial intelligence and digital platforms in enhancing blood gas analysis and preventing complications is also covered. Additionally, the chapter addresses the challenges of oxygen toxicity and acid-base imbalances during anesthesia and emphasizes the importance of early detection and intervention. The significance of postoperative blood gas monitoring in preventing respiratory failure and other complications is also discussed.

Keywords: blood gas analysis, anesthesia, arterial blood gas, venous blood gas, capnography, transcutaneous monitoring, AI in anesthesia

1. Introduction

1.1 The importance of blood gas analysis in anesthesia

Blood gas analysis is a critical method for evaluating the respiratory and metabolic status of patients during anesthesia [1]. Continuous monitoring of body functions under anesthesia is vital, particularly for assessing the adequacy of respiration and maintaining the body's acid-base balance. Arterial and venous blood gases directly reflect the patient's oxygenation status, carbon dioxide elimination, and acid-base equilibrium. Therefore, blood gas analysis serves as a fundamental tool for preventing complications and optimizing the treatment process in the perioperative period.

In addition to assessing oxygenation adequacy and ventilation effectiveness during anesthesia, blood gas monitoring is indispensable for managing acid-base imbalances [2].

IntechOpen

1.2 Blood gas monitoring: Historical development and current status

Blood gas analysis began with arterial blood gas (ABG) samples, and over time, technological advancements have allowed for faster and more reliable results. Although non-invasive methods have been developed today, arterial blood gas analysis is still considered the gold standard. However, venous blood gas (VBG) measurements are being used as an alternative monitoring method in critically ill patients, offering certain advantages. Central venous blood gas parameters are sufficiently reliable to substitute for arterial blood gas values in hemodynamically stable patients [2].

1.3 The role of blood gas values in anesthesia practices

Close monitoring of blood gas values during anesthesia plays a critical role in evaluating the patient's respiratory functions and determining ventilation strategies. Arterial blood gas (ABG) parameters are regularly measured to assess the patient's metabolic status and ensure acid-base balance during anesthesia. Conditions such as hypercapnia (high PCO_2) or hypocapnia (low PCO_2) provide important clues for optimizing respiratory management. Moreover, continuous monitoring of oxygen saturation is crucial to prevent oxygen toxicity.

Arterial blood gas analysis remains the most commonly used method to monitor the effectiveness of oxygenation and ventilation in patients under anesthesia. Although non-invasive measurement techniques are evolving, ABG is still considered the gold standard [3].

2. Methods of blood gas monitoring

2.1 Arterial blood gas analysis (ABG)

Arterial blood gas (ABG) analysis is the most commonly used method to monitor a patient's oxygenation and ventilation status during anesthesia. ABG is an invasive method performed by taking a sample directly from arterial blood, measuring levels of oxygen (PaO_2), carbon dioxide ($PaCO_2$), pH, and bicarbonate (HCO_3^-). This method provides the most accurate assessment of the patient's metabolic and respiratory condition, serving as a crucial guide in the clinical decision-making process.

Arterial blood gas (ABG) analysis is considered the gold standard for evaluating oxygenation and managing respiratory function during anesthesia [4].

2.2 Venous blood gas analysis (VBG)

Venous blood gas (VBG) analysis is used as an alternative to ABG, particularly in critically ill patients. VBG sampling is less invasive and easier to perform compared to ABG. However, venous blood gas does not accurately reflect oxygen levels. Despite this limitation, the pH and PCO_2 results from venous blood gas analysis often show good correlation with ABG, making it a reliable option in stable patients.

Central venous blood gas (VBG) analysis shows good correlation with arterial blood gas values and can be used as a less invasive alternative in critically ill patients [2] (**Table 1**).

Parameter	Arterial blood	Venous blood
PaO_2	High (80–100 mmHg)	Low (30–40 mmHg)
$PaCO_2$	Low (35–45 mmHg)	High (40–50 mmHg)
pH	Slightly higher (7.35–7.45)	Slightly lower (7.31–7.41)
Oxygen saturation (SpO_2)	High (95–100%)	Low (60–80%)

Table 1.
Clinical significance of arterial and venous blood gas differences.

2.3 Non-invasive blood gas monitoring methods

In recent years, advances in non-invasive monitoring technologies have played a significant role in evaluating a patient's respiratory functions during anesthesia [5]. Specifically, pulse oximetry allows continuous, non-invasive monitoring of the patient's oxygen saturation, enabling rapid intervention. However, methods like pulse oximetry do not fully replace blood gas measurement and require additional assessment for parameters other than oxygen saturation.

Non-invasive blood gas monitoring methods provide continuous monitoring during anesthesia but do not fully replace comprehensive blood gas analysis [3].

2.4 Clinical significance of arterial and venous blood gas differences

Arterial blood, which carries oxygen to tissues, has a high PaO_2 and a low $PaCO_2$. Venous blood, on the other hand, represents oxygen-depleted blood returning from tissues, with a lower PaO_2 and relatively higher $PaCO_2$. These differences should be considered, particularly when assessing the patient's oxygenation status and metabolic responses.

The differences between arterial and venous blood gases must be considered in clinical decision-making, especially in hemodynamically unstable patients, where these differences may be more pronounced [4, 6].

3. Blood gas parameters in anesthesia

3.1 The significance of pH, PCO2, and PO2

Maintaining safe respiratory and metabolic functions during anesthesia requires regular monitoring of blood gas parameters. The pH value is one of the most important parameters, reflecting the acid-base balance in the body. Normally ranging between 7.35 and 7.45 [7], deviations from this range lead to conditions such as acidosis or alkalosis, which may require urgent intervention in anesthesia management. PCO_2 is one of the most critical parameters indicating the effectiveness of ventilation, serving as a marker for carbon dioxide elimination. Inadequate ventilation during anesthesia can cause hypercapnia, leading to a decrease in pH (respiratory acidosis). PO_2 reflects the oxygenation status and is used to determine whether tissues are adequately oxygenated.

Measurement of arterial PCO_2 provides direct information about ventilation efficiency and is crucial for evaluating carbon dioxide elimination during anesthesia. Additionally, pH changes offer vital clues for understanding conditions like acidosis and alkalosis [2].

3.2 Acid-base balance and anesthesia

During anesthesia, especially in prolonged surgical interventions, acid-base imbalances in the patient can result in serious consequences for morbidity and mortality. Respiratory or metabolic acid-base disorders can disrupt hemodynamic stability during anesthesia. Metabolic acidosis typically arises from impaired tissue perfusion or shock, while respiratory acidosis in anesthetized patients results from inadequate ventilation [8]. Conditions such as hypercapnia and hypocapnia are among the key respiratory imbalances that must be carefully monitored during anesthesia. Excessive ventilation can lead to hypocapnia, characterized by low PCO_2, which in turn may cause alkalosis (**Table 2**).

Maintaining acid-base balance is critical for preserving hemodynamic stability during anesthesia. Both metabolic and respiratory acidosis increase the risk of complications during the perioperative period and can create situations requiring rapid intervention [2, 3].

Several clinical conditions contribute to metabolic acidosis, including diabetic ketoacidosis (DKA), dehydration, fever, and sepsis. Intoxications from substances such as tricyclic antidepressants (TCAD), opiates, cocaine, methamphetamines, salicylates, and alcohol can also cause profound acidosis. Additionally, iatrogenic causes like the overuse of normal saline in fluid resuscitation can lead to hyperchloremic metabolic acidosis. Monitoring arterial blood gas (ABG) values in these cases is crucial to detect acid-base imbalances early and guide the treatment plan, especially in the context of anesthesia management.

3.3 Hypercapnia and hypocapnia: Anesthesia management

Hypercapnia is characterized by an arterial PCO_2 level exceeding 45 mmHg, often resulting from inadequate ventilation. In patients under anesthesia, the effectiveness of mechanical ventilation must be continuously monitored. Hypercapnia can depress the respiratory center, affect brain function, and lead to cardiovascular complications, necessitating precise control of PCO_2 levels during anesthesia. Hypocapnia, on the other hand, occurs when PCO_2 falls below 35 mmHg due to excessive ventilation [9]. Hypocapnia can cause vasoconstriction and a reduction in cerebral blood flow, potentially impairing brain oxygenation and resulting in undesirable neurological outcomes (**Table 3**).

Hypercapnia is a serious condition that can lead to respiratory depression and hemodynamic instability. During anesthesia, hypocapnia may negatively impact cerebral perfusion, adversely affecting neurological functions [6].

In cases of metabolic acidosis, additional parameters such as the anion gap and osmolality/osmolarity play a vital role in diagnosis and management. A high anion gap metabolic acidosis often indicates the presence of toxins or severe metabolic

Condition	pH	PaCO$_2$	HCO$_3^-$	Clinical implication
Respiratory acidosis	Low	High	Normal/high	Inadequate ventilation, CO$_2$ retention
Metabolic acidosis	Low	Normal/low	Low	Excess acid production or bicarbonate loss
Respiratory alkalosis	High	Low	Normal/low	Hyperventilation, CO$_2$ depletion
Metabolic alkalosis	High	Normal/high	High	Bicarbonate excess or acid loss

Table 2.
Effects of respiratory and metabolic acidosis and alkalosis on blood gas parameters.

Condition	PaCO$_2$	pH	Effect	Management strategy
Hypercapnia	High	Low	Respiratory acidosis, decreased brain function	Increase ventilation, correct underlying cause
Hypocapnia	Low	High	Respiratory alkalosis, reduced cerebral blood flow	Reduce ventilation, monitor closely

Table 3.
Effects of hypercapnia and hypocapnia on blood gas parameters and management strategies.

derangements, such as in lactic acidosis or ketoacidosis. The osmolar gap is another critical measure, especially in cases of suspected toxic alcohol ingestion (e.g., ethylene glycol and methanol), where abnormal osmolality can provide early clues to diagnosis. Blood gas monitoring, in conjunction with these parameters, enhances the anesthesiologist's ability to manage complex metabolic disturbances.

3.4 Oxygen saturation and oxygen toxicity

Continuous monitoring of oxygenation during anesthesia is of great importance. Oxygen saturation (SpO$_2$) indicates whether tissues are receiving sufficient oxygen and is continuously monitored through pulse oximetry. When SpO$_2$ falls below 92%, oxygen therapy is required [10]. However, prolonged exposure to high concentrations of oxygen can result in oxygen toxicity. Oxygen toxicity, caused by the increase in free radicals, leads to cellular damage and can have severe effects, particularly on the lungs. Therefore, oxygen administration during anesthesia should be carefully regulated, and conditions that may lead to hyperoxia should be avoided.

Oxygen saturation is one of the parameters that must be continuously monitored during anesthesia. However, prolonged high-concentration oxygen therapy can lead to oxygen toxicity and cause lung damage [3].

4. Blood gas monitoring according to types of anesthesia

4.1 Blood gas monitoring in general anesthesia

General anesthesia is characterized by loss of consciousness, analgesia, muscle relaxation, and suppression of reflexes. During this process, the patient's respiratory functions must be fully managed by the anesthesia team. Blood gas analyses are crucial during general anesthesia to monitor both respiration and circulation. Arterial blood gas (ABG) analyses are considered the gold standard for evaluating the effectiveness of ventilation and the adequacy of oxygenation [11]. Continuous monitoring of parameters such as pH, PaCO$_2$, and PaO$_2$ is essential to maintain the patient's acid-base balance.

Mechanical ventilation is commonly used during general anesthesia, and its effectiveness is assessed through PaCO$_2$ levels. Hypercapnia indicates inadequate ventilation and impaired carbon dioxide elimination, while hypocapnia is often associated with overventilation and may reduce cerebral blood flow. Therefore, monitoring critical parameters like PaCO$_2$ and PaO$_2$ is mandatory to ensure effective ventilation management and cerebral perfusion. Blood gas analysis during general anesthesia is indispensable for assessing ventilation efficiency and requires continuous monitoring for proper mechanical ventilation management.

The prone position, commonly used in patients with acute respiratory distress syndrome (ARDS), can significantly improve oxygenation by enhancing ventilation-perfusion matching. Arterial blood gas monitoring is essential when patients are placed in the prone position, as changes in lung compliance and ventilation distribution can lead to improved PaO_2 levels. This positioning is often employed in cases where conventional ventilation strategies fail to maintain adequate oxygenation, and blood gas analysis helps to monitor the effectiveness of this intervention.

4.2 Blood gas monitoring in regional anesthesia

Regional anesthesia, including techniques such as spinal, epidural, or peripheral nerve blocks, involves blocking the sensation and motor function of a specific region. In regional anesthesia, patients typically retain their spontaneous respiratory function, minimizing the need for mechanical ventilation. Consequently, blood gas monitoring during regional anesthesia is less intensive. However, in some cases, particularly during prolonged surgeries, hypoxemia or hypoventilation may occur, warranting oxygenation monitoring [12].

During spinal or epidural anesthesia, the effects of the block on cardiovascular and respiratory functions must be considered. High-level spinal blocks may impact respiratory muscles, potentially leading to ventilation insufficiency. In such cases, monitoring oxygen saturation (SpO_2) and $PaCO_2$ is essential to ensure proper respiratory management [13].

While blood gas monitoring during regional anesthesia is less intensive compared to general anesthesia, the potential impact on respiratory functions must be carefully observed.

Special patient populations, such as those with chronic obstructive pulmonary disease (COPD), asthma, advanced age, or a history of chronic alcohol use, require careful blood gas monitoring during anesthesia. These patients often present with pre-existing respiratory or metabolic imbalances, such as chronic respiratory acidosis or metabolic alkalosis. Blood gas monitoring provides critical insights into their acid-base status and helps guide anesthesia management, particularly in ensuring adequate oxygenation and ventilation without exacerbating underlying conditions.

4.3 Blood gas monitoring under sedation

Sedation is a technique used to relax the patient and suppress certain reflexes during anesthesia. Depending on the depth of sedation, respiratory function may become suppressed. Light sedation typically allows spontaneous respiration, whereas deep sedation may suppress respiratory functions, necessitating ventilatory support. Under sedation, the risk of hypoventilation and oxygen desaturation increases, making it necessary to monitor oxygen saturation (SpO_2) and $PaCO_2$ [14].

Hypercapnia occurring during sedation is a critical condition requiring immediate intervention by the anesthetist. For patients unable to maintain spontaneous respiration, continuous ventilation monitoring and mechanical support, if needed, are essential. In this context, blood gas analyses play a crucial role in evaluating respiratory functions and preventing respiratory acidosis.

Blood gas monitoring during sedation requires careful attention to the risk of respiratory suppression. Ventilatory support should be provided when spontaneous respiration is lost [4].

4.4 Blood gas management during cardiopulmonary bypass

Cardiopulmonary bypass (CPB) is a procedure used in cardiac surgery where the patient's blood is oxygenated outside the body and pumped back into circulation. During this procedure, the patient's respiratory functions are bypassed, and blood gas management is entirely conducted through the bypass machine. Blood gas analyses must be continuously monitored during CPB, and parameters such as pH, $PaCO_2$, and PaO_2 must be maintained within ideal ranges [6].

Conditions such as hypocapnia and hypercapnia may develop during CPB, depending on the effectiveness and settings of the bypass machine. Metabolic acidosis and alkalosis can also be observed in blood gas monitoring during bypass. Therefore, the anesthesia team must make continuous adjustments based on blood gas analyses. High oxygen concentrations may also be applied during bypass, increasing the risk of oxygen toxicity, necessitating careful management of oxygenation levels.

Blood gas monitoring during cardiopulmonary bypass requires meticulous management, as the patient's respiratory functions are taken over by the bypass machine. Both ventilation and oxygenation must be carefully monitored, ensuring the maintenance of pH balance [3].

5. The role of blood gas monitoring in managing anesthesia complications

5.1 Respiratory failure and blood gas monitoring

One of the most serious complications that can develop during anesthesia is respiratory failure. Respiratory failure is usually associated with ventilation inadequacies, gas exchange disturbances, and circulatory problems. One of the key indicators of respiratory failure is the deterioration of PaO_2 and $PaCO_2$ levels measured through arterial blood gas (ABG) analysis. Hypoxemia (PaO_2 falling below 60 mmHg) and hypercapnia ($PaCO_2$ rising above 45 mmHg) are emergency conditions during anesthesia requiring immediate intervention. Respiratory dysfunction can also lead to acid-base imbalances, resulting in abnormal pH changes [15].

Hypoventilation during anesthesia may develop due to improperly adjusted ventilator settings, excessive use of muscle relaxants, or a decrease in the patient's spontaneous respiratory capacity. In such cases, blood gas analysis provides critical information for adjusting ventilation and optimizing respiratory support. Hypercapnia is a common complication indicating respiratory center suppression, especially in patients under general anesthesia.

Patients in extremis, particularly those suffering from acute respiratory distress syndrome (ARDS) following conditions such as pneumonia, sepsis, or pancreatitis, present unique challenges in blood gas monitoring. In these patients, severe hypoxemia and hypercapnia often occur due to compromised lung function. The management of such cases requires continuous arterial blood gas (ABG) monitoring to ensure adequate oxygenation and ventilation. ARDS often necessitates advanced interventions like mechanical ventilation, and prone positioning has shown significant benefits in improving oxygenation in these patients, which will be discussed in the following sections.

Respiratory failure can lead to serious complications during anesthesia, and arterial blood gas analysis is the most reliable guide for managing oxygenation and ventilation.

5.2 Postoperative management with blood gas monitoring

During the postoperative period, while the effects of anesthesia persist, the risk of complications remains high. Monitoring patients' respiratory functions during this time is essential. Postoperative hypoventilation is a common issue caused by surgical trauma, pain, opioid use, and residual muscle relaxant effects. In patients developing postoperative respiratory failure, arterial blood gas analysis (ABG) plays a critical role in the early diagnosis of conditions like hypercapnia and hypoxemia. Furthermore, opioids used for postoperative pain management may depress the respiratory center, leading to respiratory acidosis.

Postoperative blood gas monitoring ensures that patients' respiratory functions are adequately assessed until they fully recover from anesthesia. Rising $PaCO_2$ levels may indicate the need for ventilation support, while declining PaO_2 levels may require adjustments to oxygen therapy. Continuous monitoring of oxygen saturation during the postoperative period is also essential for determining oxygen needs.

Postoperative blood gas monitoring plays a critical role in early detection of complications and optimizing ventilation [16].

5.3 Acid-base imbalance and clinical intervention

One of the most common complications encountered during anesthesia is acid-base imbalance. Acidosis and alkalosis disrupt the body's normal homeostatic balance and can lead to serious clinical consequences. Respiratory acidosis occurs due to the accumulation of carbon dioxide as a result of ventilation inadequacies, leading to a decrease in arterial pH. In this case, immediate ventilation improvement is required to ensure carbon dioxide elimination. Metabolic acidosis usually arises from impaired tissue perfusion, shock, or severe bleeding. Blood gas analysis during anesthesia provides critical information for managing metabolic acidosis.

Alkalosis is often associated with excessive ventilation or metabolic disorders. Respiratory alkalosis is characterized by excessively low $PaCO_2$ levels, typically caused by hyperventilation. In such cases, reducing ventilation and restoring carbon dioxide levels to balance is necessary. Metabolic alkalosis during anesthesia is often linked to electrolyte imbalances and is managed based on blood gas analysis findings [17].

Acid-base imbalances during anesthesia can disrupt hemodynamic and respiratory stability. Blood gas analyses are critical for early detection of acid-base imbalances and determining appropriate intervention strategies [4, 11].

6. Future approaches and new technologies

6.1 Innovations in blood gas monitoring technologies

Technological advancements in blood gas analysis have contributed to safer and more efficient management of anesthesia practices. The invasive and time-consuming nature of traditional arterial blood gas (ABG) analysis has driven the development of new non-invasive methods and continuous monitoring technologies. Today, methods like transcutaneous blood gas monitoring have made significant strides in reducing the need for ABG. This technology offers an alternative by continuously measuring carbon dioxide (PCO_2) and oxygen (PO_2) levels through the skin, providing a less invasive option for blood gas analysis. Transcutaneous sensors also offer more dynamic management during surgery due to their continuous monitoring capabilities [18].

Another important innovation is the development of capnography technology. Capnography, which measures the carbon dioxide levels in exhaled gases during respiration, offers a rapid and non-invasive method for evaluating ventilation effectiveness during anesthesia. Technological improvements in capnography have facilitated the early detection of ventilation insufficiencies, helping prevent potential complications during anesthesia (**Figure 1**).

Transcutaneous blood gas monitoring and advanced capnography systems play a crucial role in clinical decision-making by providing continuous and non-invasive monitoring during anesthesia [6, 11].

6.2 Digital blood gas monitoring and remote monitoring systems

The acceleration of digitization in healthcare has led to significant changes in anesthesia management as well. Digital blood gas monitoring systems enable real-time monitoring of blood gas parameters during anesthesia, allowing these data to be analyzed through digital platforms. These systems not only provide monitoring but also facilitate the early detection of potential complications through big data analytics and artificial intelligence (AI)-supported decision support systems. Automatic detection of sudden changes in blood gas parameters and alerting the anesthesiologist plays a critical role in preventing complications.

Remote monitoring systems, on the other hand, extend the ability to monitor anesthesia applications outside the operating rooms and intensive care units. These systems allow for the remote monitoring and analysis of patients' blood gas data, enabling the management of complications from a broader perspective. Known as

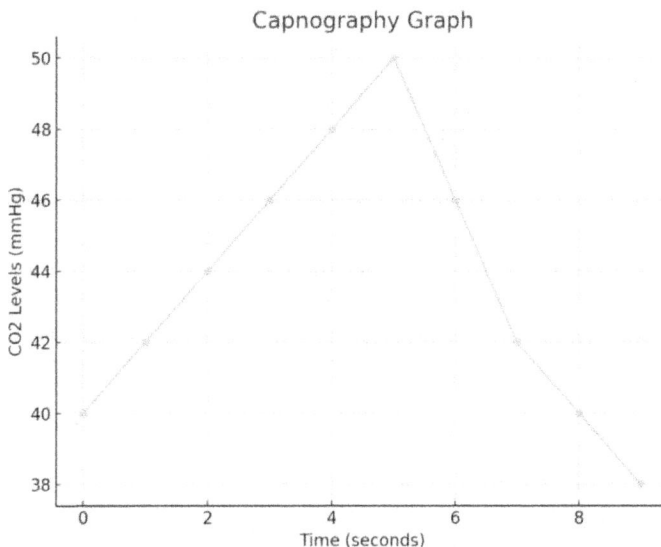

Figure 1.
Capnography graph showing the changes in CO_2 levels during the respiratory cycle. The x-axis represents time in seconds, and the y-axis represents the CO_2 levels in mmHg. During exhalation, CO_2 levels rise steadily, peaking before rapidly dropping during inhalation, illustrating the normal pattern of carbon dioxide exchange in the lungs. This graph is a key tool in evaluating ventilation efficiency during anesthesia.

telemetric monitoring, this method enhances patient safety by transmitting data collected during anesthesia to a centralized control room, reducing response time.

When combined with big data analytics and AI-supported solutions, digital blood gas monitoring and telemetric systems offer revolutionary innovations in anesthesia management [19].

6.3 AI-supported blood gas analysis

The integration of artificial intelligence (AI) technologies into healthcare has brought significant advancements in blood gas analysis. AI-supported systems can analyze large datasets, detect abnormal changes in blood gas parameters during anesthesia, and develop personalized treatment strategies based on this data. AI-powered algorithms automate the monitoring of parameters such as pH, $PaCO_2$, PaO_2, and HCO_3^-, offering more precise and faster results compared to manual assessments.

AI is also utilized not only for data analysis but also for treatment recommendations. AI-based clinical decision support systems can optimize ventilation settings or determine the need for additional oxygen therapy based on changes in the patient's blood gas parameters during anesthesia. The potential of AI in this area is considered an important step toward enhancing patient safety by minimizing human error during anesthesia.

AI-supported blood gas analysis, combined with big data analytics and clinical decision support systems, allows for the implementation of more personalized and safer treatment strategies during anesthesia [20].

7. Conclusion

Blood gas monitoring during anesthesia plays a critical role in safely and effectively managing patients' respiratory and metabolic functions. Arterial blood gas (ABG) and venous blood gas (VBG) analyses provide anesthesiologists with vital information about patients' ventilation, oxygenation, and acid-base balance. Complications that may develop under anesthesia can be detected early through accurate and continuous monitoring of blood gas parameters, enabling the development of appropriate intervention strategies.

In addition to traditional arterial blood gas analysis, non-invasive methods such as transcutaneous blood gas monitoring, capnography, and pulse oximetry offer easier monitoring by minimizing the risks associated with invasive procedures. However, despite the speed and convenience offered by non-invasive methods, they still cannot fully match the accuracy provided by arterial blood gas analysis. This highlights that ABG remains the gold standard, particularly in the management of critically ill patients.

Technological advancements are bringing significant innovations to anesthesia management. Artificial intelligence (AI)-supported systems and big data analytics have the potential to optimize clinical decision-making by detecting changes in blood gas parameters more precisely and quickly during anesthesia. Digital blood gas monitoring systems and remote tracking applications enhance patient safety and enable the early prevention of complications. These innovations allow anesthesiologists to develop more personalized, data-driven treatment strategies.

Blood gas monitoring is crucial not only during anesthesia but also in the postoperative period. Postoperative complications such as respiratory failure, acid-base imbalances, and hypoventilation can be detected early through regular blood gas monitoring, positively impacting post-anesthesia care processes.

Blood gas monitoring during anesthesia is critical for managing both intraoperative and postoperative complications, and with digitalization, more effective monitoring methods are being offered.

In conclusion, blood gas monitoring continues to be one of the cornerstones of safety in anesthesia practices. With the integration of technological developments and innovations like artificial intelligence, blood gas monitoring methods are becoming more secure and efficient, minimizing complications. It is anticipated that these technologies will be more widely used in the future, bringing further advancements to anesthesia practice.

Acknowledgements

The author acknowledges the usage of ChatGPT 4.0 for the language improvement of the text.

Author details

Semin Turhan
Department of Anesthesiology and Reanimation, Hitit University Erol Olçok Training and Research Hospital, Çorum, Turkey

*Address all correspondence to: smnondr@hotmail.com

IntechOpen

References

[1] Gray S, Powell LL. Blood gas analysis. In: Burkitt-Creedon JM, Davis H, editors. Advanced Monitoring and Procedures for Small Animal Emergency and Critical Care. Chichester: John Wiley & Sons, Ltd; 2012. pp. 286-292

[2] Chong WH, Saha BK, Medarov BI. Comparing central venous blood gas to arterial blood gas and determining its utility in critically ill patients: Narrative review. Anesthesia and Analgesia. 2021;**133**(2):374-378

[3] Raemer DB, Francis D, Philip JH, Gabel RA. Variation in PCO_2 between arterial blood and peak expired gas during anesthesia. Anesthesia and Analgesia. 1983;**62**(12):1065-1069

[4] Wade RG, Crawfurd J, Wade D, Holland R. Radial artery blood gas sampling: A randomized controlled trial of lidocaine local anesthesia. Journal of Evidence-Based Medicine. 2015;**8**(4):185-191. DOI: 10.1111/jebm.12177

[5] Folke M, Cernerud L, Ekström M, Hök B. Critical review of non-invasive respiratory monitoring in medical care. Medical and Biological Engineering and Computing. 2003;**41**:377-383

[6] Ailawadi G, Zacour RK. Cardiopulmonary bypass/extracorporeal membrane oxygenation/left heart bypass: Indications, techniques, and complications. Surgical Clinics. 2009;**89**(4):781-796

[7] Onyekwelu AC, Abdullahi HI, Isah AY, Jamda AM, Nwegbu MM. Ionised serum calcium reference interval among rural women of reproductive age in Abuja, Nigeria. The Nigerian Postgraduate Medical Journal. 2021;**28**(1):39-43

[8] Bonhomme V, Demoitie J, Schaub I, Hans P. Acid-base status and hemodynamic stability during propofol and sevoflurane-based anesthesia in patients undergoing uncomplicated intracranial surgery. Journal of Neurosurgical Anesthesiology. 2009;**21**(2):112-119

[9] Holla VV, Prasad S, Pal PK. Neurological effects of respiratory dysfunction. Handbook of Clinical Neurology. 2022;**189**:309-329

[10] Gottlieb J, Capetian P, Hamsen U, Janssens U, Karagiannidis C, Kluge S, et al. German S3 guideline: Oxygen therapy in the acute care of adult patients. Respiration. 2022;**101**(2):214-252

[11] Georges M, Rabec C, Monin E, Aho S, Beltramo G, Janssens JP, et al. Monitoring of noninvasive ventilation: Comparative analysis of different strategies. Respiratory Research. 2020;**21**:1-10

[12] Ehrenfeld JM, Funk LM, Van Schalkwyk J, Merry AF, Sandberg WS, Gawande A. The incidence of hypoxemia during surgery: Evidence from two institutions. Canadian Journal of Anaesthesia. 2010;**57**(10):888

[13] Pusapati RN, Sivashanmugam T, Ravishankar M. Respiratory changes during spinal anaesthesia for gynaecological laparoscopic surgery. Journal of Anaesthesiology Clinical Pharmacology. 2010;**26**(4):475-479

[14] Fu ES, Downs JB, Schweiger JW, Miguel RV, Smith RA. Supplemental oxygen impairs detection of hypoventilation by pulse oximetry. Chest. 2004;**126**(5):1552-1558

[15] Witting MD, Lueck CH. The ability of pulse oximetry to screen for hypoxemia and hypercapnia in patients breathing room air. The Journal of Emergency Medicine. 2001;**20**(4):341-348

[16] Fogagnolo A, Montanaro F, Al-Husinat LI, Turrini C, Rauseo M, Mirabella L, et al. Management of intraoperative mechanical ventilation to prevent postoperative complications after general anesthesia: A narrative review. Journal of Clinical Medicine. 2021;**10**(12):2656

[17] Tinawi M. Respiratory acid-base disorders: Respiratory acidosis and respiratory alkalosis. Archives of Clinical and Biomedical Research. 2021;**5**(2):158-168

[18] Rithalia SV. Developments in transcutaneous blood gas monitoring: A review. Journal of Medical Engineering and Technology. 1991;**15**(4-5):143-153

[19] Singh M, Nath G. Artificial intelligence and anesthesia: A narrative review. Saudi Journal of Anaesthesia. 2022;**16**(1):86-93

[20] Schweiger G, Malorgio A, Henckert D, Braun J, Meybohm P, Hottenrott S, et al. Visual blood, a 3D animated computer model to optimize the interpretation of blood gas analysis. Bioengineering. 2023;**10**(3):293

Chapter 4

Mathematical Modeling of Oxygen and Carbon Dioxide Exchange in Hollow Fiber Oxygenators

Lal Babu Khadka, Foivos Leonidas Mouzakis, Ali Kashefi,
Johannes Greven, Khosrow Mottaghy and Jan Wilhelm Spillner

Abstract

Artificial lungs are commonly used in cardiopulmonary-bypass surgery (CPB), extracorporeal life support (ECLS), and extracorporeal carbon dioxide removal therapy (ECCO2R). In this study, a semi-empirical model for O_2 and CO_2 transfer in an oxygenator was formulated to evaluate the gas exchange performance at different blood/gas flow rates and various inlet conditions. The model uses experimentally obtained mass transfer coefficients together with blood-gas and acid-base inlet parameters to determine the corresponding outlet values by considering the mass transfer equations for both O_2 and CO_2. Increasing the blood flow rate (1–7 L/min) decreases pO_2 at the outlet (from 376 to 120 mmHg), but linearly increases the total oxygen transfer rate (OTR) from 76 to 450 mL/min. CTR, the CO_2 transfer rate (64–648 mL/min), depends primarily on the ratio of gas to blood flow rate (1:1–5:1). In addition, venous concentrations of O_2–CO_2 play a pivotal role in the overall gas exchange efficiency of the oxygenator. Conclusively, a good agreement (R^2=0.99) could be observed between the experimental data and the model's predictions for OTR and CTR alike at standard inlet conditions. The model's capabilities can be extended by modeling gas exchange during CPB, ECLS and ECCO2R therapies for different connection configurations.

Keywords: oxygenator, semi-empirical model, mass transfer, blood-gas analysis, *in vitro*, gas exchange

1. Introduction

An oxygenator is a medical device used in extracorporeal lung support therapy as an artificial lung. There are three basic designs of oxygenators: bubble oxygenators, thin-film oxygenators, and membrane oxygenators [1]. Currently, a microporous hollow fiber membrane oxygenator is the universally accepted standard design for gas exchange during cardiopulmonary-bypass (CPB), extracorporeal life support systems (ECLS), or extracorporeal carbon dioxide removal therapy (ECCO2R). It consists of thousands of microporous hollow micro-fibers that are

IntechOpen

bundled together within a polymer case [2]. The capillaries are usually made of polymethylpentene (PMP), silicone, or polypropylene (PP) [3]. Membrane oxygenation prevents the direct physical contact between gas and blood phases and minimizes blood trauma. It also requires lower priming volumes compared to other designs. However, it also significantly increases the resistance of the permeating gas species due to the formation of a laminar boundary layer, an impedance that critically hampers gas exchange between the two phases [4, 5]. The physical dimensions of an oxygenator depend on the manufacturing process and the target patients. For example, a commercial oxygenator for adults such as MEDOS HILITE® 7000 has a surface area of 1.9 m^2 and 310 mL of priming volume, whereas the neonatal variant (MEDOS HLITE® 1000) has a surface area of 0.39 m^2 and a priming volume of 57 mL [6]. **Figure 1** depicts the gas exchange occurring in a typical hollow fiber oxygenator, where blood and gas flow in countercurrent directions. Here, gas flows inside the fiber lumen while blood courses in the open space between the hollow fibers. The countercurrent flow pattern maintains the pressure gradient of oxygen and carbon dioxide between blood and gas phases along the entire length of the oxygenator and optimizes the overall gas transfer rate. A heat exchanger is often integrated in the oxygenator, or annexed to the circuit to regulate the temperature of blood within the physiological range (37 ± 1°C).

The general performance of an oxygenator is evaluated by calculating the oxygen transfer rate (*OTR*) and carbon dioxide transfer rate (*CTR*) at different blood and gas flow rates. **Table 1** lists the blood inlet conditions to evaluate the *OTR* and *CTR* of an oxygenator according to contemporary standards (ISO 7199/2016) [7]. The naturally occurring *OTR* and *CTR* of an average person is around 250 mL/min and 200 mL/min, respectively [8].

Here, a semi-empirical mathematical model was formulated for the estimation of oxygen and carbon dioxide transfer taking place in a commercial hollow fiber

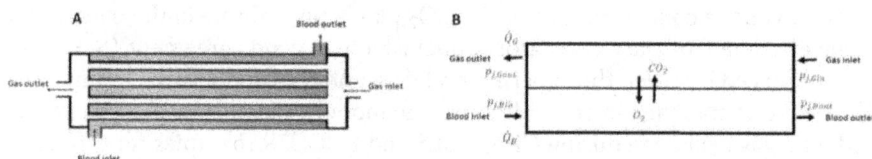

Figure 1.
(A) General design of hollow fiber oxygenators with countercurrent blood and gas flows. Blood uptakes oxygen, and its saturation increases as it flows toward the outlet. (B) Inlet and boundary conditions: blood & gas flow rates and partial pressure of the individual gas species at the respective inlet-outlet ports (j = [O$_2$, CO$_2$]).

Parameters	Range
Oxyhemoglobin saturation	60 ± 5%
Base excess	0 ± 5 mmol/L
pCO$_2$	45 ± 5 mmHg
Hb	12 ± 1 g/dL
Temperature	37 ± 1 °C

Table 1.
Inlet condition required for testing oxygenator performance according to ISO 7199/2016 [7].

oxygenator based on the principle of conservation of mass and on mass transfer equations. The performance of the oxygenator at standard inlet conditions was first evaluated according to AAMI: ISO 7199:2016, and the mass transfer coefficients for both oxygen and carbon dioxide were determined. The parameters obtained were then fed into the numerical model simulating the oxygenator to extrapolate the acid-base and blood-gas parameters at diverse inlet conditions (e.g., gas flow/blood flow ratios, partial pressure of oxygen, and carbon dioxide at the inlet).

2. Methodology

Assessment of the oxygenator's gas exchange performance and the subsequent estimation of the mass transfer coefficients of oxygen and carbon dioxide was accomplished via *in vitro* investigations with fully heparinized porcine blood in accordance with AAMI: ISO 7199:2016 standard. The inlet conditions for the experiment are provided in **Table 1**. The fundamental components constituting the experimental setup have been previously described by Khadka et al. [9]. The role of the test apparatus was assumed by an adult oxygenator with 1.95 m^2 surface area and a priming volume of 320 mL. Blood flow rate was monitored by an ultrasonic flowmeter (Transonic, Ithaca, NY, USA), whereas gas flowmeters (Platon, Vienna, Austria) were utilized for the regulation of gas supply. **Figure 2** displays the test setup.

Pre-and post-oxygenator (i.e., venous and arterial) blood samples were drawn at frequent intervals to be analyzed with a blood-gas analyzer (Radiometer, Copenhagen, Denmark). The blood-gas analyzer's (BGA) report of each sample included

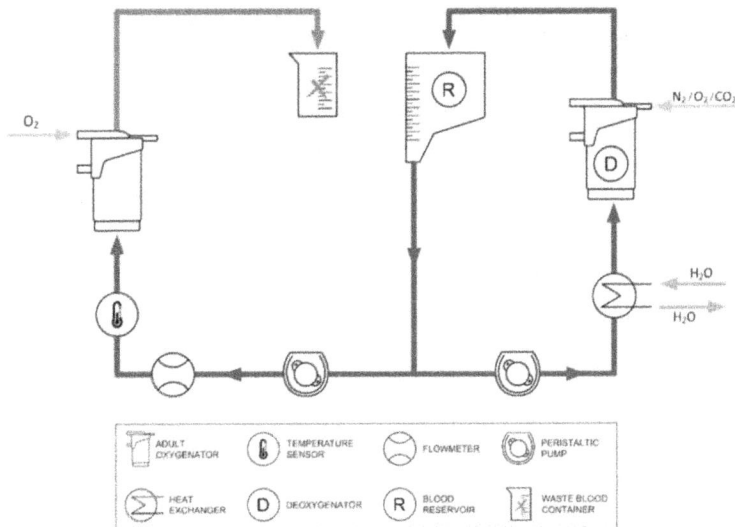

Figure 2.
Graphical representation of the experimental setup. The circuit consists of two adult oxygenators (one performs as a deoxygenator), two peristaltic pumps, a heat exchanger, and a blood reservoir. In terms of sensors: blood flow is monitored via a liquid flowmeter, whereas gas supply is regulated via three gas flowmeters. A temperature sensor guarantees that blood temperature remains within 37 ± 1°C, while a pressure gauge keeps track of the inlet and outlet pressure of the test oxygenator. The blue and red lines indicate venous and arterial (saturated) blood, respectively.

diverse parameters such as the partial pressure of oxygen (pO_2) and carbon dioxide (pCO_2), oxygen saturation (S), the respective concentration of both gases in blood, c_{O_2} and c_{CO_2}, along with pH, bicarbonate concentration (HCO_3^-), hemoglobin concentration (Hb), Hematocrit value (Hct), atmospheric pressure (p_{atm}), etc. These values were implemented in the calculation of the experimental OTR and CTR.

For the mathematical model, the concentration of carbon dioxide in plasma ($c_{CO_2,p}, mL/L$) and in whole blood ($c_{CO_2}, mL/L$) was estimated from its partial pressure ($pCO_2, mmHg$) and pH using the Henderson-Hasselbalch and Douglas equations [10, 11] as shown below (Eqs. (1)–(4)).

$$pH = 6.1 + \frac{[HCO_3^-]}{[0.03pCO_2]} \tag{1}$$

$$[HCO_3^-] - H_i = m(pH - pH_i) \tag{2}$$

$$c_{CO_2,p} = 22.26 . \alpha_{CO_2} . pCO_2 . 10^{pH - pK} \tag{3}$$

$$c_{co_2} = c_{co_2,p}\left(1 - \frac{0.0289 c_{Hb}}{(3.352 - 0.00456.S(\%))(8.142 - pH)}\right) \tag{4}$$

α_{CO_2} and pK are 0.0307 $mmol/L/mmHg$ and 6.0907 respectively. H_i and pH_i are the initial bicarbonate concentration and pH, and m is the slope of the buffer line equation.

Similarly, oxygen saturation (S) and concentration ($c_{O_2}, mL/L$) were calculated from its partial pressure ($pO_2, mmHg$) using the simplified Hill equation [12] as given in Eqs. (5)–(7). Where 32.558, 0.266 and 2.9 are the experimentally derived parameters for porcine blood, 1.34 mL_{O_2}/g_{Hb} is the Hüfner constant, and $\alpha_{O_2} = 0.00317\ mL_{O_2}/dL$ is the solubility coefficient of oxygen at 37°C. Hb (g/dL) is the hemoglobin concentration in blood, and Hct (%) is the hematocrit value, which is considered to be three times that of the Hb.

$$S = 100 \frac{1 + \left(\frac{pO_2}{pO_{2,50}}\right)^{2.9}}{\left(\frac{pO_2}{pO_{2,50}}\right)^{2.9}} \tag{5}$$

$$pO_{2,50} = 32.558 . 10^{0.266\ (\ln(40) - \ln(pCO_2))} \tag{6}$$

$$c_{O_2} = 10\left[1.34.Hb.\frac{S(\%)}{100} + \alpha_{O_2}pO_2\left(1 - \frac{Hct}{100}\right)\right] \tag{7}$$

Gas exchange in an oxygenator is depicted in **Figure 1**. Nitrogen, N_2, flowrate is considered negligible in comparison to O_2 and CO_2 flowrate. Total gas flow rate is assumed to be constant throughout the length of the oxygenator ($\dot{Q}_{G,in} \approx \dot{Q}_{G,out} \approx \dot{Q}_G$). The partial pressure of water vapor, p_{H_2O}, is 0 $mmHg$ at the gas inlet and 47 $mmHg$ at the gas outlet. p_{atm} and $pO_{2,Gin}$ are around 747 $mmHg$, and $pCO_{2,Gin}$ is 0 $mmHg$.

Mass transfer equation for oxygen,

$$OTR = \dot{Q}_G\left(\frac{pO_{2,Gin}}{p_{atm}} - \frac{pO_{2,Gout}}{p_{atm} - p_{H_2O}}\right) \tag{8}$$

$$OTR = \dot{Q}_B(c_{O_2,Bout} - c_{O_2,Bin}) \tag{9}$$

$$OTR = k_{O_2} A_{oxy} \frac{(pO_{2,Gout} - pO_{2,Bin}) - (pO_{2,Gin} - pO_{2,Bout})}{ln\left(\frac{pO_{2,Gout} - pO_{2,Bin}}{pO_{2,Gin} - pO_{2,Bout}}\right)} \tag{10}$$

Mass transfer equation for carbon dioxide,

$$CTR = \dot{Q}_G\left(\frac{pCO_{2,Gout}}{P_{atm} - P_{H_2O}}\right) \tag{11}$$

$$CTR = \dot{Q}_B(c_{CO_2,Bin} - c_{CO_2,Bout}) \tag{12}$$

$$CTR = k_{CO_2} A_{oxy} \frac{pCO_{2,Bout} - (pCO_{2,Bin} - pCO_{2,Gout})}{ln\left(\frac{pCO_{2,Bout}}{pCO_{2,Bin} - pCO_{2,Gout}}\right)} \tag{13}$$

OTR and *CTR* are the oxygen and carbon dioxide transfer rates (mL/min), p is the partial pressure in $mmHg$, $c_j \, mL_j/L_{blood}$ is the concentration of species j (O_2 or CO_2) in blood, $\dot{Q}_G(mL/min)$ and $\dot{Q}_B$ (L/min) are the gas and blood flow rates in the oxygenator, and k_j ($mL_j/(min.m^2.mmHg)$) is the total mass transfer coefficient of species j (O_2 or CO_2). Subscript G is for gas, B is for blood, *in* is for inlet, and *out* is for outlet. A_{oxy} is the total surface area of the oxygenator. k_{O_2} and k_{CO_2} at different blood flow rate were calculated using the data from **Tables 2** and **3**.

Eqs. (8)–(13) are six non-linear equations with six unknowns: *OTR*, *CTR*, $pO_{2,Bout}$, $pO_{2,Gout}$, $pCO_{2,Bout}$ and $pCO_{2,Gout}$. The final equations are solved in Python programming language using SciPy package. The effect of gas and blood flow rate on pO_2 and pCO_2 at the outlet, and the overall *OTR* and *CTR* of the oxygenator were calculated for different combinations of gas flow/blood flow ratios (1:1, 2:1, 5:1) and inlet $pO_{2,Bin}$ (25, 30, and 40 mmHg).

3. Results

Table 2 summarizes the partial pressure of oxygen and oxygen saturation at the inlet and outlet of the oxygenator as obtained from the *in vitro* experiment with porcine blood. The average pO_2 and S at the inlet is 41.5 $mmHg$, and 63.3%, respectively. The relationship between kO_2 and $\dot{Q}_B$ is shown in **Figure 3**.

Q_B [L/min]	Inlet		Outlet		OTR [mL/min]	kO_2 [mL/min. mmHg.m^2]
	pO_2[mmHg]	S [%]	pO_2[mmHg]	S [%]		
1	41.81 ± 1.41	63.8 ± 0.98	465.11 ± 79.20	99.66 ± 0.49	62.95 ± 2.24	0.078 ± 0.01
3	41.81 ± 1.41	63.8 ± 0.98	340 ± 105.46	99.63 ± 0.52	188.02 ± 6.93	0.20 ± 0.03
5	41.82 ± 1.30	63.5 ± 0.88	227.11 ± 60.92	98.68 ± 0.30	396.12 ± 6.97	0.28 ± 0.02
7	40.63 ± 1.84	62.06 ± 2.62	130.80 ± 31.54	97.43 ± 0.92	428.94 ± 22.8	0.36 ± 0.02

Table 2.
OTR and kO_2 at different Q_B. Hb, inlet pO_2, and pCO_2 are 12.9 g/dL, 747 mmHg, and 45 mmHg, respectively. The inlet and outlet values for pO_2 and S are obtained experimentally by measuring the blood-gas and acid-base parameters via BGA. OTR increases linearly with rising blood flow rate.

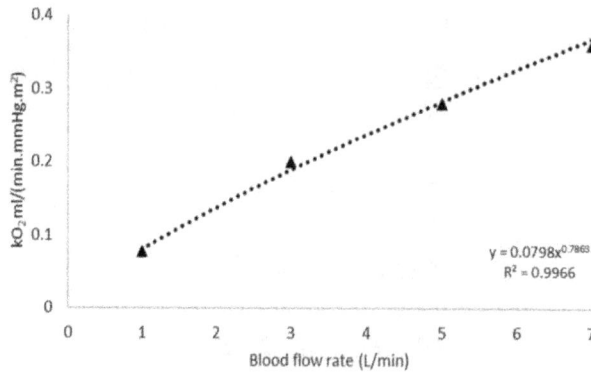

Figure 3.
Mass transfer coefficient of oxygen at different blood flow rates. An increase in blood velocity decreases the thickness of the boundary layer, resulting in reduced gas exchange resistance and an elevated mass transfer coefficient.

Similarly, the partial pressure of carbon dioxide and *pH* at the inlet and the outlet of the oxygenator, along with *CTR* and the carbon dioxide mass transfer coefficient at different $\dot{Q}_B$ are shown in **Table 3**. **Figure 4A** depicts the relationship between kCO_2

$\dot{Q}_B$ [L/min]	Inlet		Outlet		CTR [mL/min]	kCO_2 [mL/min. mmHg.m^2]
	pCO_2 [mmHg]	pH	pCO_2 [mmHg]	pH		
1	47.29 ± 1.27	7.367 ± 0.004	23.78 ± 0.49	7.550 ± 0.005	136.15 ± 3.70	9.5 ± 0.6
3	47.29 ± 1.27	7.367 ± 0.004	28.38 ± 0.59	7.499 ± 0.005	331.65 ± 12.6	10 ± 0.67
5	47.40 ± 1.34	7.376 ± 0.003	31.83 ± 0.33	7.479 ± 0.007	460.56 ± 25.32	10.33 ± 0.73
7	46.23 ± 1.03	7.380 ± 0.007	33.5 ± 0.51	7.459 ± 0.006	553 ± 26.19	11.12 ± 0.81

Table 3.
CTR and kCO_2 at different $\dot{Q}_B$. Hb, $pCO_{2,Gin}$ and $\dot{Q}_G$: $\dot{Q}_B$ are 12.9 g/dL, 0 mmHg, and 2:1, respectively. The inlet and outlet values for pCO_2 and pH are obtained experimentally by measuring the blood-gas and acid-base parameters via BGA. CTR also increases linearly with blood flow rate.

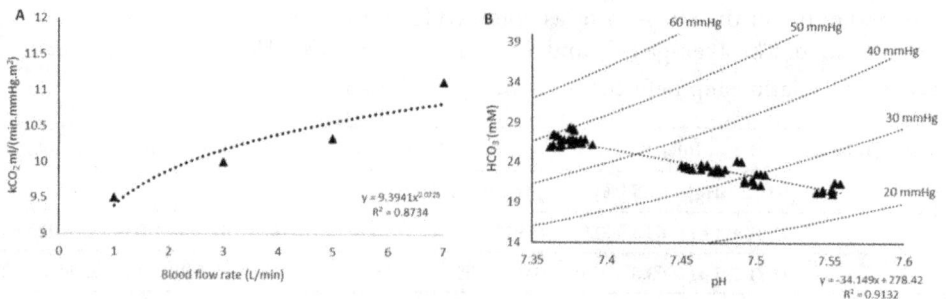

Figure 4.
(A) Relationship between kCO_2 and $\dot{Q}_B$. The mass transfer coefficient of CO_2 is markedly higher than that of oxygen and only increases slightly with an increase in blood flow rate. (B) pH vs. HCO_3^- diagram depicting the change in pH during the removal of carbon dioxide for a change in pCO_2 between approx. 60 mmHg to 20 mmHg. The linear relationship between bicarbonate concentration and pH is depicted via the buffer line equation. This buffer line indicates the direction of respiratory compensation for a pH change due to extracorporeal CO_2 elimination. The slope of the buffer line (−34.149) depends primarily on Hb concentration.

and $\dot{Q}_B$. The effect of carbon dioxide elimination on pH during the experiment is shown in **Figure 4B**, in the pH vs. HCO_3^- diagram.

The experimentally obtained data for oxygen and carbon dioxide were fitted to the mathematical model in the corresponding Eqs. (8)–(13). **Table 4** summarizes the values predicted by the semi-empirical model for $pO_{2,Bout}$, $pCO_{2,Bout}$ S, OTR and CTR for the inlet values of $pO_{2,Bin} = 40$ mmHg, $pCO_{2,Bin} = 45$ mmHg, $Hb = 12.9$ g/dL, $\dot{Q}_B =$ 1–7 L/min and $\dot{Q}_G/\dot{Q}_B = 2:1$.

Figure 5A–D depicts the numerically estimated output predicted by the semi-empirical model for different input conditions. For all the inlet $pO_{2,Bin}$ variations (25 mmHg, 30 mmHg, 40 mmHg), the outlet $pO_{2,bout}$ decreases constantly with blood flow rate (**Figure 5A**). Furthermore, the outlet saturation also depends on the initial saturation of venous blood (30, 42, 62%), thus affecting the oxygen transfer rate

$\dot{Q}_B$ [L/min]	pO_2 [mmHg]	S [%]	pCO_2 [mmHg]	OTR [mL/min]	CTR [mL/min]
1	376.87	99.94	24.55	75.59	131.16
3	224.72	99.72	27.92	211.15	316.427
5	154.88	99.12	30.46	335.74	438.28
7	120.45	98.12	32.39	450.23	524.12

Table 4.
Oxygen and carbon dioxide transfer rates and their respective partial pressures at the outlet of the oxygenator as predicted by the numerical model. Inlet $pO_{2,Bin}$, $pCO_{2,Bin}$ and $\dot{Q}_G/\dot{Q}_B$ are 40 mmHg, 45 mmHg and 2:1, respectively. Both OTR and CTR increase linearly with blood flow rate. The numerically generated values for OTR and CTR show high correlation ($R^2 = 0.99$) with the experimental values.

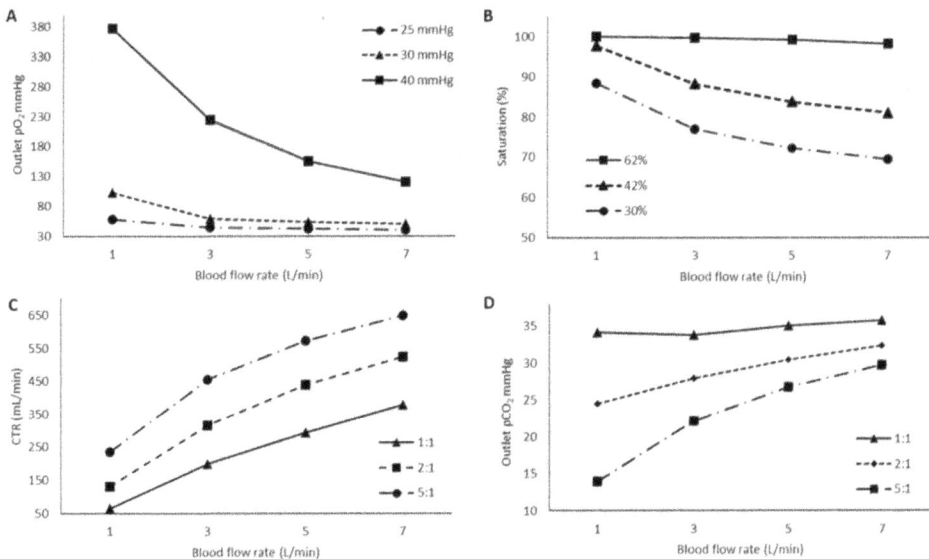

Figure 5.
(A) $pO_{2,Bout}$ at different $pO_{2,Bin}$ (25, 30 and 40 mmHg) as estimated from the mathematical model. $pCO_{2,Bin}$ is 45 mmHg. The $pO_{2,Bout}$ decreases with increasing blood flow rate for any $pO_{2,Bin}$. (B) Oxygen saturation at the outlet for different inlet saturations (30%, 42% and 62%). $pCO_{2,Bin}$ is 45 mmHg. (C) CTR at different $\dot{Q}_G/\dot{Q}_B$ (1:1–5:1). $pO_{2,Bin}$ and $pCO_{2,Bin}$ are 40 mmHg and 45 mmHg, respectively. CTR increases linearly with $\dot{Q}_B$ for constant $\dot{Q}_G/\dot{Q}_B$. (D) $pCO_{2,Bout}$ at different $\dot{Q}_G/\dot{Q}_B$ (1:1–5:1). $pO_{2,Bin} = 40$ mmHg and $pCO_{2,Bin} = 45$ mmHg. Hb is 12.9 g/dL in every case.

(**Figure 5B**). Similarly, the carbon dioxide transfer rate, CTR, is dependent both on gas and blood flow rate (**Figure 5C and D**), as it increases linearly with $\dot{Q}_B$ for all the provided $\dot{Q}_G/\dot{Q}_B$ ratios (1:1–5:1) (**Figure 5C**).

4. Discussion

Using the mass transfer and mass conservation principles for oxygen and carbon dioxide, a semi-empirical numerical model of an artificial lung has been developed as an addendum to the mathematical model introduced by Khadka et al. [9] in order to consider the gas exchange phenomena in an oxygenator. The new version differentiates itself from the older one in the implementation of a modified Hill equation with experimentally derived parameters for the numerical estimation of oxygen concentration from its partial pressure in furtherance of minimizing the margin of error.

The mass transfer coefficients of oxygen and carbon dioxide of the oxygenator were determined using experimental data obtained from *in vitro* investigations with porcine blood (**Tables 2 and 3**), which were fed afterward into the semi-empirical model to assess the theoretical performance of the oxygenator at different inlet blood-gas values and acid-base states. The obtained carbon dioxide transfer coefficient is significantly higher than that of oxygen due to the high solubility of carbon dioxide in blood compared to oxygen. However, the resistance to gas diffusion decreases at higher blood flow rates due to the deflating boundary layer [13], resulting in elevated mass transfer coefficients for both oxygen and carbon dioxide (**Figures 3 and 4A**).

The findings of the numerical simulation suggest that blood flow rate has a higher impact on the partial pressure of oxygen at the blood outlet and its overall oxygen transfer rate. Arterial pO_2 decreases monotonously from 376 mmHg to 120 mmHg with increasing blood flow rates (1–7 L/min), for inlet pO_2 of 40 mmHg (**Table 4**). That being said, oxygen saturation in venous blood plays a significant role in the oxygen transfer rate and directly affects the saturation levels at the outlet. In a hypoxic patient with venous saturation of around 42%, for instance, saturation at the outlet of the given oxygenator stays below 85% at higher blood flow rates ($\geq$ 5 L/min) (**Figure 5B**). However, oxygenators with higher surface area or embellished mass transfer coefficients are capable of delivering outlet saturations well above 95% at higher blood flow rates ($\geq$ 5 L/min), even when inlet saturation is lower than 42%.

Elimination of carbon dioxide by means of an oxygenator increases the *pH* of blood along the buffer line as **Figure 4B** denotes. The slope of the buffer line is determined by the total hemoglobin concentration in the blood.

In general, carbon dioxide removal chiefly depends on the gas flow / blood flow ratio [14]. As **Figure 5C** indicates, doubling the gas flow rate offers nearly 50% increase in carbon dioxide elimination (292 vs. 438 mL/min), whereas a fivefold increase of gas flow / blood flow ratio can yield CTR values enhanced by 95% at a constant blood flow rate of 5 L/min (292 vs. 570 mL/min). Both oxygen and carbon dioxide transfer rates increase linearly with rising blood flow rates at constant gas flow / blood flow ratios.

To realize the gas transport modeling several assumptions had to be made. Utilization of the aforementioned simplified mass transport equations for countercurrent flows was accomplished under the hypothesis of a steady state solution with purely convective transport. It was also theorized that the oxygen-hemoglobin reaction remained always in equilibrium, and that the total gas flow rate remained constant over the entire length of the hollow fibers. Blood flow was also considered to be homogeneous throughout the oxygenator. Additionally, metabolic compensation was also not taken into account for acid-base balance, despite the fact that during an *in vivo* application, metabolic compensation could cause a shift in the buffer line.

Such simplifications may affect the overall accuracy of the model and limit its applicability when used in an *in vivo* setting. Furthermore, the model has been validated so far only with porcine blood. Therefore, further experiments with human blood are necessary for the optimization of the relevant parameters, prior to any clinical implementation.

Ultimately, the introduced mathematical model of an artificial lung has been conceived with a single purpose in mind: the ability to emulate the gas exchange performance of any commercially available oxygenator *in silico*. The disclosed results corroborate this statement, and the fact that the numerically derived values for OTR and CTR correlate highly (R^2 = 0.99) with the experimental data further emphasize the model's potential as a valuable tool for the assessment of gas exchange in diverse therapies (e.g., CPB, ECMO, and ECCO2R) and different connections. Complex models can be evaluated by devising the corresponding *in vitro* circuits mimicking these connections [15].

5. Conclusion

A mathematical model of an oxygenator capable of evaluating the gas transfer between countercurrent flows across hollow fibers was established on experimentally derived mass transfer coefficients for oxygen and carbon dioxide. The exchange of oxygen and carbon dioxide and its impact on acid-base balance was estimated based on the combined transfer rate formulas for oxygen and CO_2 along with the Henderson-Hasselbach, Douglas, and modified Hill equations. The obtained numerical results correlate highly with the experimental data in standard settings. Hence, the model is capable of determining the performance of any oxygenator at diverse blood/gas flow rates and inlet conditions (e.g., acid-base balance) not only in terms of gas exchange but also by predicting the blood-gas and acid-base parameters at the outlet. In future, the model will be integrated into the mathematical of a cardiopulmonary system for the estimation of oxygen and carbon dioxide exchange during complex procedures such as CPB, ECLS, and ECCO2R. Eventually, this could become an indispensable tool assisting in decision-making by determining the influence of different operating conditions (blood-gas flow rates, oxygenator size, connection type, etc.) on the overall oxygen and carbon dioxide transfer rate during such therapies.

Conflict of interest

The authors declare no conflict of interest.

Author details

Lal Babu Khadka[1], Foivos Leonidas Mouzakis[1*], Ali Kashefi[1], Johannes Greven[2], Khosrow Mottaghy[1] and Jan Wilhelm Spillner[2]

1 Medical Faculty, Institute of Physiology, RWTH Aachen University, Aachen, Germany

2 Medical Faculty, Department of Thoracic Surgery, RWTH Aachen University, Aachen, Germany

*Address all correspondence to: lal.babu.khadka@rwth-aachen.de

IntechOpen

References

[1] Holman WL, Timpa J, Kirklin JK. Origins and evolution of extracorporeal circulation: JACC historical breakthroughs in perspective. JACC. 2022;**79**:1606-1622. DOI: 10.1016/j.jacc.2022.02.027

[2] Suma K, Tsuji T, Takeuchi Y, Inoue K, Shiroma K, Yoshikawa T, et al. Clinical performance of microporous polypropylene hollow-fiber oxygenator. The Annals of Thoracic Surgery. 1981;**32**:558-562. DOI: 10.1016/S0003-4975(10)61798-5

[3] Ting H, Songhong Y, Jinhui H, Dejian C, Jie L, Hongjun H, et al. Membranes for extracorporeal membrane oxygenator (ECMO): History, preparation, modification and mass transfer. Chinese Journal of Chemical Engineering. 2022;**49**:46-75. DOI: 10.1016/j.cjche.2022.05.027

[4] Iwahashi H, Yuri K, Nosé Y. Development of the oxygenator: Past, present, and future. Journal of Artificial Organs. 2004;**7**:111-120. DOI: 10.1007/s10047-004-0268-6

[5] Costa AM, Halfwerk FR, Thiel JN, Wiegmann B, Neidlin M, Arens J. Effect of hollow fiber configuration and replacement on the gas exchange performance of artificial membrane lungs. Journal of Membrane Science. 2023;**680**. DOI: 10.1016/j.memsci.2023.121742

[6] Medos Hilite. Oxygenation Systems for Adults, Paediatrics and Infants. 2024. Available from: https://kategorizacia.mzsr.sk/Pomocky/Download/RequestAttachment/29508 [Accessed: June 16, 2024]

[7] ISO 7199:2016. Cardiovascular Implants, and Artificial Organs—Blood-Gas Exchangers (Oxygenators). Geneva, Switzerland: ISO; 2016

[8] Komoda T, Matsunaga T. Biochemistry of internal organs. In: Biochemistry for Medical Professionals. London: Academic Press, Elsevier; 2015. pp. 65-73. DOI: 10.1016/B978-0-12-801918-4.00005-0

[9] Khadka LB, Mouzakis FL, Kashefi A, Hima F, Spillner JW, Mottaghy K. Blood gas parameters and acid–base balance during extracorporeal lung support with oxygenators: Semi-empirical evaluation. Mathematics. 2023;**11**:4088. DOI: 10.3390/math11194088

[10] Constable PD. Acid-base assessment: When and how to apply the Henderson-Hasselbalch equation and strong ion difference theory. The Veterinary Clinics of North America. Food Animal Practice. 2014;**30**:295-316. DOI: 10.1016/j.cvfa.2014.03.001

[11] Douglas AR, Jones NL, Reed JW. Calculation of whole blood CO2 content. Journal of Applied Physiology. 1985;**1988**(65):473-477. DOI: 10.1152/jappl.1988.65.1.473

[12] Annesini MC, Marraelli L, Piemonte V, Turchetti L. Blood oxygenators and artificial lungs. In: Artificial Organ Engineering. 1st ed. London: Springer-Verlag; 2017. pp. 117-157

[13] Mostafavi AH, Mishra AK, Ulbricht M, Denayer JFM, Hosseini SS. Oxygenation and membrane oxygenators: Emergence, evolution and Progress in material development and process enhancement for biomedical applications. Journal of Membrane Science and Research. 2021;**7**:230-259. DOI: 10.22079/JMSR.2021.521505.1431

[14] Manap HH, Wahab AKA, Zuki FM. Mathematical modelling of carbon dioxide exchange in hollow fiber membrane oxygenator. In: IOP Conference Series: Material Science and Engineering. 2017. p. 210. DOI: 10.1088/1757-899X/210/1/012003

[15] Hima F, Kalverkamp S, Kashefi A, Mottaghy K, Zayat R, Strudthoff L, et al. Oxygenation performance assessment of an artificial lung in different central anatomic configurations. The International Journal of Artificial Organs. 2023;**46**(5):295-302. DOI: 10.1177/03913988231168163

Chapter 5

A New Approach to Understanding Diabetic Retinopathy from Retina Vessels Blood SaO₂ Study

Luis Niño-de-Rivera, Erwin Michel Davila-Iniesta and Félix Gil-Carrasco

Abstract

This chapter discusses a new method for assessing SaO₂ oxygen saturation from fundus photography (EFP). In addition, a new method for assessing SaO₂ oxygen saturation from fundus photography (EFP) is discussed. These enhancement differences follow the evolution of ocular diseases associated with metabolic dysfunctions in which the oxygen saturation SaO₂ plays a key role. A new visual and numerical method to follow the evolution of diabetic retinopathy, glaucoma, or other degenerative eye diseases is also discussed. The chapter shows how the fundus photograph of the eye (EFP) is segmented to show its oxygen content from each pixel of the EFP. In this chapter, we discuss the description of ocular SaO₂ as a mathematical function that allows us to understand measurable differences in the metabolic output of blood within the retinal microvasculature. The SaO₂ function across the ocular microvasculature system is a set of numbers that can be analyzed using statistics or other mathematical tools to better understand the complex metabolic process within the ocular microvasculature system. The chapter will show graphical and analytical results of healthy eyes compared to the disease diabetic retinopathy. It is hoped that this new approach will allow the clinician to better understand the evolution of diabetic eye disorders.

Keywords: diabetic retinopathy, eye fundus photography (EFP), fundus images, oxygen saturation (SaO₂), optical coherence tomography (OCT), retinal microvasculature, retinal oximetry, retinal vessel segmentation

1. Introduction

Diabetic retinopathy (DR) is one of the most important causes of visual loss worldwide and is the leading cause of vision impairment in patients with diabetes, with an estimated 130 million people with the disease by 2030 and 161 million by 2045 [1]. DR is usually asymptomatic until the advanced stages. To prevent further visual loss and disease progression, it is necessary to regularly monitor patients with diabetes and ensure awareness of the metabolic disturbances that they undoubtedly present in the retinal microvasculature [1, 2].

DR analyses from conventional sightseeing Eye Fundus Photography (EFP) images and optical coherence tomography (OCT) are not enough to understand correctly the complex metabolic process in the retinal microvasculature [1, 2]. Traditional methods are based on the physician's clinical experience, and even the clinic's expertise always welcomes a better approach to joining technology with new image processing tools, database platforms from optical coherence tomography, and artificial intelligence, which will improve physicians' labor.

The human retina is one of the most demanding oxygen systems in the human body. The retina, to ensure health, requires a continuous supply of oxygen through its microcirculatory system [3]. Retinal ischemia is undesired to any degree since it leads to vision loss. Clinicians do not have efficient methods to measure the evolution of ischemia in degenerative eye illness. Diabetic retinopathy and glaucoma, by their clinician manifestation, supposes insufficient oxygen in the retina blood system [4]. However, there are non-invasive facilities to follow properly ischemia. Under that scope, we discuss new alternatives to evaluate Oxygen Saturation SaO_2 from EFP, an essential non-invasive procedure.

Non-invasive retinal oximetry is constantly developed to find more precise oxygenation measurements from retinal veins since invasive methods to measure $SaO2$ inside the ocular globe are unavailable. Physicians will surely enjoy looking at the retina vessel size, arterial, and vein structure, thickness, and blood color differences associated with $SaO2$ to follow illness performance. $SaO2$ evaluation is a critical issue in monitoring eye degenerative diseases [3–5]. However, photo oximetry faces essential challenges in evaluating SaO_2 inside the retinal circulatory system. Among others, photo oximetry requires efficient segmentation methods to properly separate the arterial and vein retina complex structures to show oxygen consumption through the eye's circulatory system. Eye fundus images require proper image processing procedures to expose blood color differences associated with blood SaO_2. The hemoglobin Hb has the highest blue tone, if nonoxygen carries in there. In contrast, the highest red tone is for the oxyhemoglobin HbO_2, with the highest levels of oxygen in the arterial system [3–6]. The effect of wavelength looking at the same EFP image after segmentation and color assignment is shown below.

This research aims to show researchers and physicians new alternatives to follow SaO_2 performance in different stages of the illness. The SaO_2 performance in the retina circulatory system is represented numerically as a set of pixels whose value has a linear relationship with its oxygen content, and then the SaO_2 map represents a matrix which value sequences is a mathematical function. The disease is seen not only as a set of symptoms, but also as a numerical description of ocular metabolic dysfunction and a mathematical function was found to describe how the O_2 process works in ocular degenerative diseases such as diabetic retinopathy or any other pathology related to O_2 deficiencies (**Figure 1**).

1.1 The light absorbance complexity

The incidence and reflectance of light at the ocular globe face complex non-linear light absorption phenomena related to the wavelength of the emitting light camera sensor. The blue and red graph in **Figure 2** shows the absorbance coefficient of Hb and HbO_2 when exposed to incident light from 300 to 1000 nanometers (nm). The Blue Hb graph represents blood with cero O_2, which means oxygen saturation at cero %, $SatO_2 = 0$, while the red graph HbO_2 represents arterial blood with maximum O_2 content, $SaO_2 = 100$.

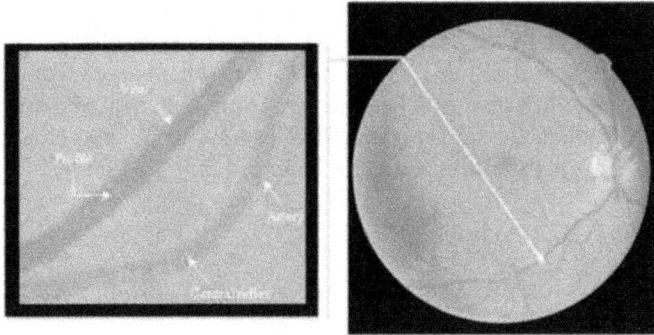

Figure 1.
Example of the different color shades between veins and arteries from images taken with specialized cameras where the different thicknesses between the two corpora cavernosa are visualized. Fundus images show sensitivity in the central area of light reflection in retinal arteries and veins [7].

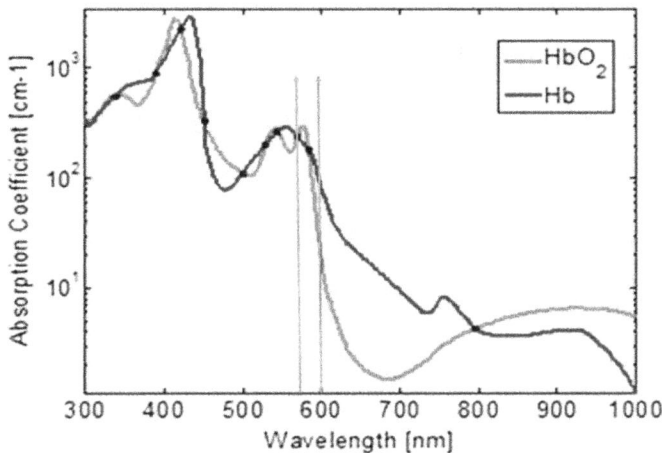

Figure 2.
Shows the Hb and HbO₂ light Absorption Coefficient AC when blood is exposed to wavelengthWL from 300 to 1000 nanometers (nm). The Blue Hb graph represents blood with cero O₂ content, while the red graph HBO₂ represents arterial blood with 100% of saturated O₂.

Wavelength plays a vital role in EFP image acquisition. As shown in **Figure 2**, Hb and HbO$_2$ have the same absorbance coefficient at 540, 570, and 800 nm. This supposes the same scale reference to measure the light reflected from veins and arterials when an incident light goes through them. However, at 600 nm, the absorbance coefficient is lower for HbO$_2$, about one order of magnitude with respect to Hb. At first sight, 540 and 570 nm. are the optimum wavelengths for analyzing SaO$_2$, assuring the same energy is reflected for both arterial and venues. However, the frequency at 600 nm finds the absorbance coefficient one order of magnitude lower than at 570 nm [3, 4, 6].

The incident light at a wavelength of 600 nm will reflect more of the red tones of HbO$_2$ than the blue tones of Hb. At 802 nm, the absorption coefficient is the same for both HbO$_2$ and Hb, and it is the lowest absorption coefficient for both HbO$_2$ and Hb [3].

It is stated that at 802 nm, the absorption coefficient is the same for both HbO$_2$ and Hb, with the lowest absorption coefficient. This makes 802 nm a favorite wavelength for getting the highest possible tone intensity reflected in the image with very similar scale tone tonality for both venues and the arterial system. Furthermore, it is important to look at any EFP and acquire conciseness about what we see from EFP coming from different wavelength images. The same eye from EFP from 570 nm and 600 nm will not necessarily show the same retina vessel system, as shown below.

A deeper discussion about this topic can be found in Refs. [3–6].

1.2 A brief look at retinal oximetry

The importance of the wavelength has already been mentioned; let us briefly look at the parameters of the EFP eye sensor. The Lambert–Beer law lets us calculate the intensity of light transmitted through a solution. According to Eq. (1), the Lambert–Beer law shows the relationship between the intensity of light I transmitted through solutions and the intensity of incident light Io [3, 8]. The light I transmitted through the blood depends on three variables: two of them related to blood chemistry: its extinction coefficient (molar absorbance) of the blood sample (ε) and its hematocrit concentration (c), and a third one that depends on the distance through the sample (d) or path length (d) of the optic system (**Figure 3**).

$$I = I_0 e^{-cd\varepsilon} \tag{1}$$

I = Intensity of light transmitted through the sample.

Io = Incident light intensity (light intensity before interaction with the sample).

The optical density (OD) shows the relationship between transmitted light I and the incident light I_0 [9–11]. in blood. This relationship ($-\log_{10}(I/I_0)$) is a linear dependency of (ε*c*d).

$$\mathrm{ODlog10I}/I_0) = \left(\varepsilon^* c^* d\right) \tag{2}$$

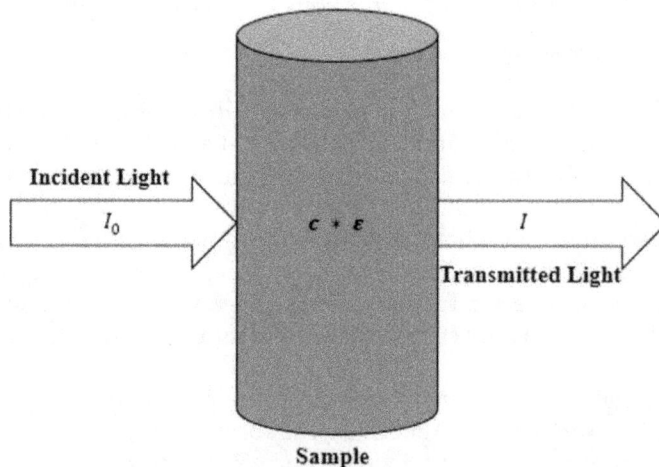

Figure 3.
Graphical representation of incident light ray I_0, transmitted light ray I, concentration of the absorbing substance c, the molar absorption coefficient ε and the optical path length d.

However, the light absorbance of a blood sample at any given wavelength is called lambda optical density ($OD\lambda$) and is defined as:

$$OD\lambda = \log\frac{I}{I0} = \varepsilon * c * d. \tag{3}$$

There is an isosbestic wavelength where the extinction coefficients for Hb and HbO$_2$ are identical. Then, in this case, the OD for blood depends only on c, d. However, at a non-isosbestic wavelength, the extinction coefficients for Hb and HbO$_2$ are different, and the OD depends on c d and oxygen saturation [9]. The ratio between two ODs at two distinct wavelengths, one isosbestic and the other non-isosbestic, ODR is sensitive to oxygen saturation [10]:

$$ODR = \frac{OD\ Non - isobestic}{OD - isobestic} \tag{4}$$

2. Methodology

Based on the above discussion, a set of tools is available to assess SaO$_2$ using numerical and graphical tools. The aim of this research work is to apply this methodology to images of healthy and diseased cases and to look for numerical differences to aid in the diagnosis and monitoring of the disease and to focus on finding differences in SatO$_2$ in Diabetic Retinopathy DR not only by a visual image showing SaO$_2$ performance but also by a numerical vector of SaO$_2$ to allow the researcher or clinician a better understanding of the metabolic dysfunction in DR disease.

2.1 Oxygen calculus of the blood

The Blood Oxygen Saturation SaO$_2$ is the relationship between HbO$_2$ and (HbO$_2$ + Hb), as discussed in [2]:

$$SatO_2 = \frac{HbO_2}{HB + HbO_2} * 100\% \tag{5}$$

This straightforward relation will give the percentage of HbO$_2$ compared with the oxygen in both HbO$_2$ + Hb [3, 6]. SatO$_2$ computing in Eq. (1) requires the same relative scale for both Hb and HbO$_2$, like in 540 and 570 nm; however, the absorbance coefficient for Hb and HbO$_2$ is different at most wavelengths, as shown in **Figure 2**. The oxygen saturation equation, according to Eq. (1), requires an adjustment for image wavelengths where the absorbance coefficient is not the same, non-isosbestic such as 418, 542, 577, and 925 nm, where HbO$_2$ has the highest absorption points, and 430, 550, 758, and 910 nm, where Hb has its highest absorption values.

$$SatO_2 = a(ODR) + b \tag{6}$$

where a and b are constants. Karlsson et al. [8] reports a = −1.28 and b = 1.24.

Arteries and veins in EFP reflect different gray tonalities [7] depending on wavelengths and optics parameters. The oxygen, seen from EFP gray images, considers the gray tonality changes proportional to O_2 on venues and arteries. The first gray level (1/255) in the 1 to 255 is the absence of O_2 in Blood. Each of the 255 levels represents 0.39% of $SatO_2$. The gray level 255 means a pixel full of oxygen, with 100% of $SatO_2$ (0.39 × 255 = 100) [3].

The performance of $SatO_2$ in the circulatory eyeball system (COGS) can be easily shown by its gray hue ranging from (1 to 255), but also equivalent from purple to red, transforming the gray to red, green, and blue RGB. This approach considers each pixel as HbO_2 cumulus representation, delivering oxygen through its way until HbO_2 loses O_2 to become Hb with 1 to 50 levels. The vessels, HbO_2, Hb, and consequently, its oxygen content are filtered by a segmentation process, becoming the circulatory eye system into a numerical matrix that represents its oxygen content, estimated by $SatO_2$ and represented by a set of gray tones or its translation to RGB to show an EFP colored image.

The set of gray colors in Hb and HbO_2 is a numeric vector that graphically shows the metabolic process's performance. Physicians can see the evolution of the illness from segmented EFP more precisely from a set of numbers than from typical OCT or eye fundus images, where diagnosis depends on the physician's expertise, always a man's subjective interpretation.

2.2 Pseudocolor tonality map

The Pseudocolor Tonality Map shows the O_2 transition from HbO_2 to Hb. The deoxyhemoglobin Hb is the set of levels at the gray scale from 0 to 187 corresponding to tonalities in RGB going from purple, blue, and green, equivalent to 30–70% of $SatO_2$.

The $SatO_2$ from 71–100% is the set of gray levels going from 188 to 255, which, converted to RGB, shows $SatO_2$ as colors going from yellow to red. Veins and arterial color transition is a visual representation of $SatO_2$ performance. The $SatO_2$ is easily computed from number 0 to 255 by $SatO_2$ = (number)*(0.39) (**Figure 4**).

Figure 5A shows a healthy eye from HRF database [12]. **Figure 5B** shows the segmented and colored EFP according to Equation. **Figure 5B** separates the O_2 concentration by a set of colors. The red represents O_2 concentration going from the

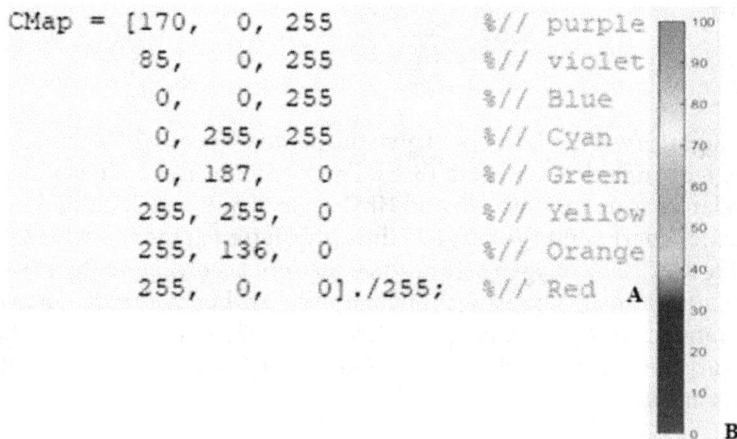

```
CMap = [170,   0, 255        %// purple        100
         85,   0, 255        %// violet         90
          0,   0, 255        %// Blue           80
          0, 255, 255        %// Cyan           70
          0, 187,   0        %// Green          60
        255, 255,   0        %// Yellow         50
        255, 136,   0        %// Orange         40
        255,   0,   0]./255;  %// Red      A    30
                                                20
                                                10
                                             0  B
```

Figure 4.
(A) shows the colorimetric proposal of the pseudo color to show (B) the oxygen transition from Hb to HbO_2.

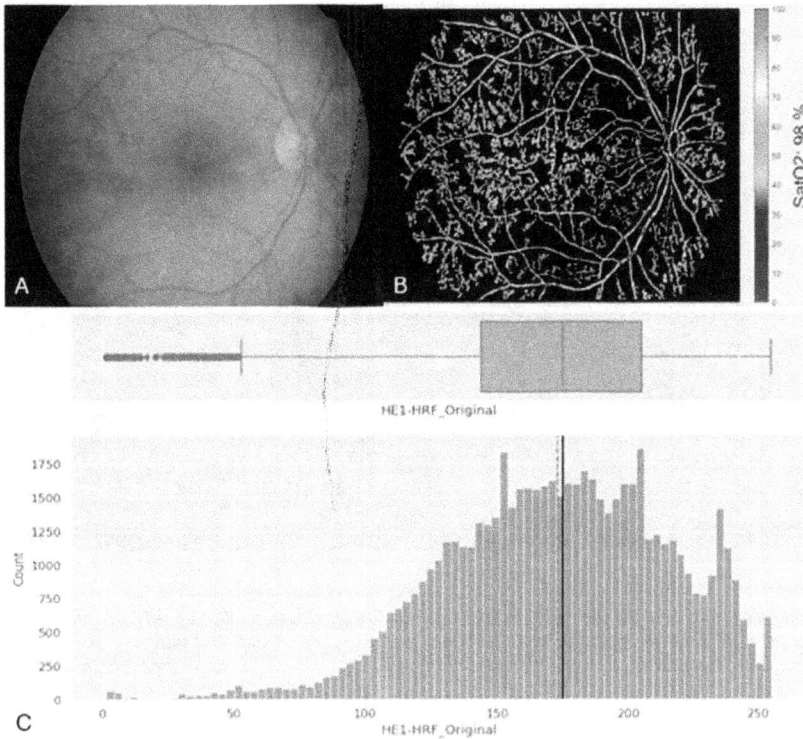

Figure 5.
(A) shows the original image from the HRF database [12], (B) shows the colorimetric proposal of the pseudo color for the original image and (C) shows the oxygen concentration depending on the gray level intensity of the image (A).

highest red tone to the lowest, as red loses O$_2$ in yellow, green, and blue end violet. **Figure 5C** shows the amount of accumulated O$_2$ by gray level, count versus oxygen concentration in the 1 to 255 scale. This count versus SatO$_2$ on a 0 to 255 scale is the estimation of O$_2$ distribution through microvasculature. This objective set of values allows comprehensive mathematical analysis of what is going on with O$_2$ performance inside the retina microvasculature. This is the counterpart of the subjective interpretation from conventional EFP analysis.

The oxygen yield in the microvasculature tree can be further analyzed. In **Figure 6A**, we show the EFP microvasculature extracted from **Figure 5A**, which shows all gray levels. **Figure 6B** shows pseudo color EFP with a pixel tonality from 0 to 95. **Figure 6C** shows the O$_2$ distribution from 96 to 199; this is the green zone representing the O$_2$ lost transition, and **Figure 6D** shows the reds with the highest content of O$_2$ from 200 to 255.

2.3 The light absorption in the blood a practical case

This section presents the effects of isosbestic and non-isosbestic wavelengths on the same image after EFP segmentation and pseudocolor assignment. First, the absorbance coefficient must be correctly understood when using an isosbestic wavelength; then, the results are compared by applying the SatO$_2$ algorithm, proposed in this work, to the same EFP image at 570 nm and 600 nm [4, 9–11]. **Figure 7B** on the left shows the EFP Oxymap T1 at 570 nm from Kristjánsdóttir et al. [10].

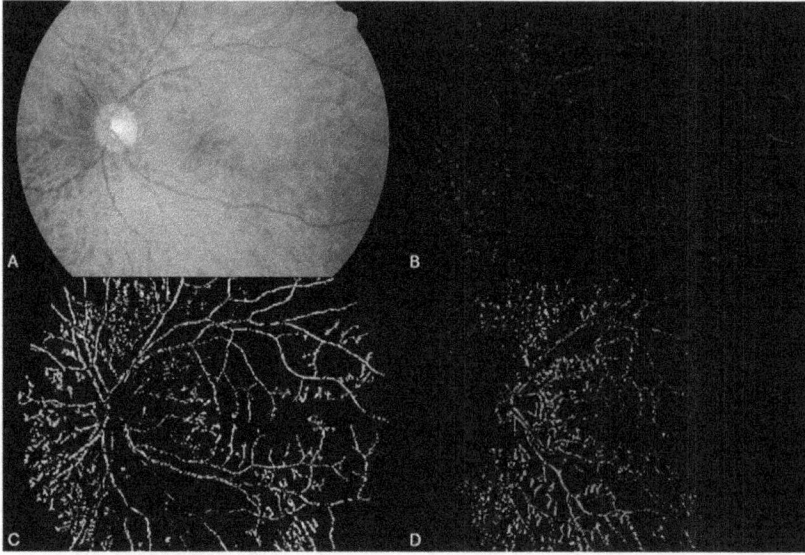

Figure 6.
Shows the O_2 performance in the microvasculature separated by three sets of color tonality. (A) shows the original image from the HRF database [12], (B) shows the areas where oxygen saturation is minimal, (C) shows the areas where oxygen saturation exists but is not the maximum, and (D) shows the areas where the highest amount of oxygen saturation is found.

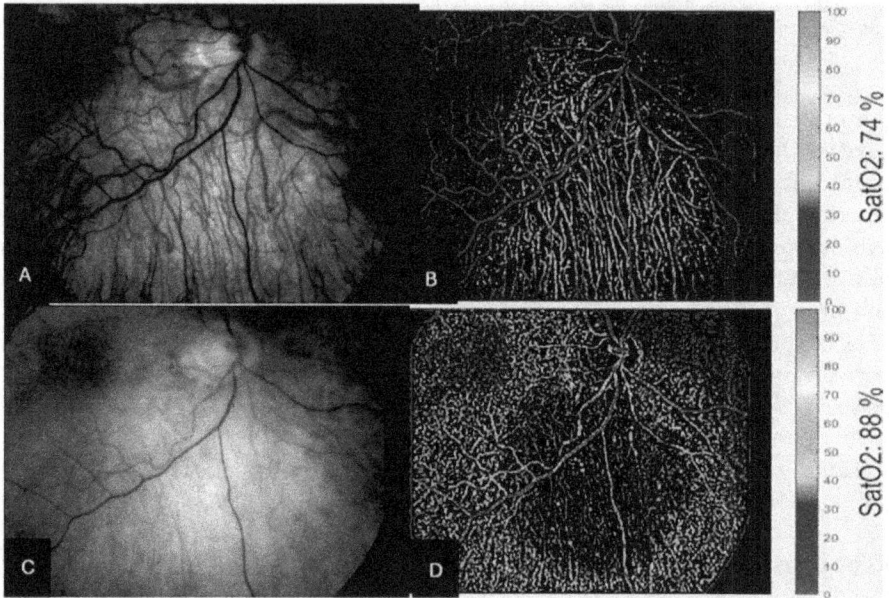

Figure 7.
The veins and arterial systems at 570 and 600 nm, obtained by Kristjánsdóttir et al. [10] using Oxymap T1, ensure the same scale hue for both veins and arterial colorimetry. (A) shows the image obtained at 570 nm by Kristjánsdóttir. (B) shows the application of the pseudo color method applied to (A). (C) shows the image obtained at 600 nm by Kristjánsdóttir. (D) shows the application of the pseudo color method to (C).

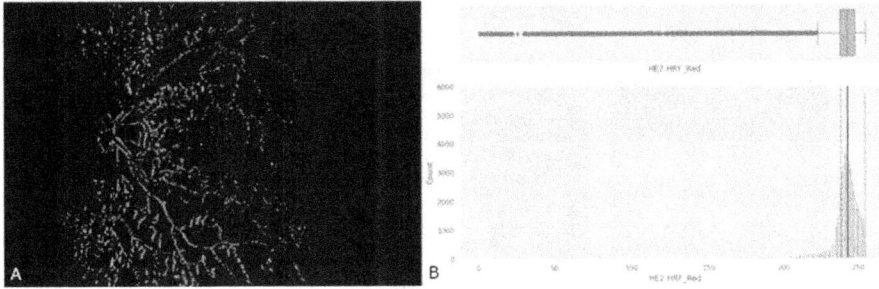

Figure 8.
(A) shows the zone where reds are distributed in the arterial tree. Red intensities are proportional to its SaO_2.
(B) shows how many pixels are in each level from 198 to 255. This is called the Oximetric function distribution.

Figure 7B at left shows a healthy gray eye fondus image taken from Oxymap T1 at 570 nm. **Figure 6C** at left shows the same image but taken at 600 nm, both images reported by Kristjánsdóttir et al. [9], in their important work that discusses Oxymap T1 tune and software $SatO_2$ visual sight associated with OxymapT1. On the right in **Figure 7B**, oxygen saturation in veins and arterial branches is shown using the color tone method [3].

The reader must distinguish the arterial network difference from the venue system from 570 to 600 nm. As said above, at 570 nm, light reflectance is the same for both HbO_2 and Hb, which means that oxygen reflectance is proportionally the same for arterial and venue systems; this proportionality is not detectable by sight at the original image. It can be seen in the colored image how, at 600 nm, the absorption coefficient enhances the arterial network (HbO_2) because it is an order of magnitude higher than Hb. This schematically shows that wavelength plays a vital role in SaO_2 analysis. The strategy of representing SaO_2 as a vector allows it to be examined separately, which means that the regions from 200 to 255 can be processed as the set of points and zones with the highest O_2 levels. This idea is in **Figure 7**, which shows the zone where reds are distributed in the arterial tree. Red intensities are proportional to its $SatO_2$, which shows how many pixels are in each level from 198 to 255 in the saturation function graph. This is called the oximetric function distribution. **Figure 8B** shows the distribution of O_2 count by gray level. This means if there are 255 at 255 level, there are 255-pixel cells with 100 of SaO_2.

3. Results

3.1 Healthy cases

The oxygen saturation estimates of the healthy eyes have an oxygen saturation percentage of 93% ± 7%, where the eye with the lowest oxygen saturation has a value of 85%, while the eye with the highest oxygen saturation percentage has a value of 98%.

Seventeen EFR images of healthy eyes with the optic nerve oriented to the right were selected from the database used by Cen et al. [13] to apply the pseudocolor method discussed above. **Table 1** shows the results of the first four images analyzed. The reader can find all the processed images from that database together with the codes used to obtain the results shown at https://github.com/MetatronEMDI/Fundus-Images-Results.

Table 1.
Application of the pseudo color method applied to patients HE-1 to HE-4 (Healthy Eye [13]). In addition to the graphing of the repetition of the values obtained from the vector of each image.

Table 1 shows that the arterial and venue trees are clearly defined over a black background, showing a clear sclera by contrast. The count function associated with each EFP shows a similar going-up tendency from the lowest value to its mean value (1 to 50) and a similar download from its mean to near 200. **Figure 9** shows the comparative density performance of the 17 $SatO_2$ eyes. It is observed that the highest SaO_2 pattern, the (200 to 255) curve that compares the SaO_2 performance of the 17 healthy eyes, has the same approach in the red range. It looks like a rectifier sine wave with a mean value in the valley's middle. This pattern was found to remain constant in red tones for healthy eyes.

3.2 Diabetic retinopathy analysis by $SatO_2$ performance

This section discusses the results from our $SatO_2$ pseudocolor method applied to a set of Diabetic Retinopathy DR cases to look for new tools. Diabetic retinopathy is classified as Diabetic Retinopathy Type 1 DR1, Diabetic Retinopathy Type 2 DR2, and Diabetic Retinopathy Type 3 DR3. The study analyzes sets of DR1, DR2, and DR3 EFP images previously classified by traditional methods. These analyses show colorimetry $SatO_2$ performance in the retina microvasculature system for each DR. In addition,

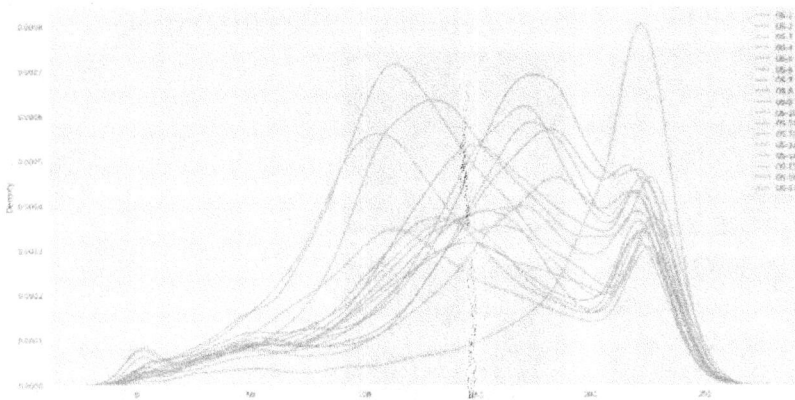

Figure 9.
Shows the comparative density performance of the 17 $SatO_2$ eyes.

the oximetry density function is the key to finding numerical singularities among Diabetic Retinopathy status. The differences among DR1, DR2, and DR3 are measurable, as shown in the result below. The methodology used to analyze DR performance is the same as the one discussed above for healthy eyes.

3.2.1 Diabetic retinopathy type 1

DR grading from Hammersmith [14] evaluates five components of retinopathy: microaneurysms and hemorrhages, exudates, new vessels, venous irregularities, and retinitis proliferating. Those five issues are highly related to retina microvasculature changes. A new approach to help recognize those variables is $SatO_2$ performance from EFP images. This DR1 analysis uses 11 EFP images previously classified as DR1 from a public database used by Cen et al. [13]. All images have the optic nerve oriented to the right. **Table 2** shows four DR-1-EFP images after segmentation and colored by our method. The reader can analyze the 11 DR1 images from the next link (https://github.com/MetatronEMDI/Fundus-Images-Results). Notice from the link that it is not evident from the original EFP images that those are DR1. However, colorimetry shows images 2, 6, 7, 8, 9, 10, and 11 have more green areas than red ones. $SatO_2$ estimations are not conclusive since all of them are 93% ± 7%. **Table 1** shows a clear tendency to lose $SatO_2$. The DR1 $SatO_2$ density distribution function tends to increase lower O_2 values with a decrease in the red region (200 to 255) (**Figure 10**).

Table 2 shows four DR1 EFP images after segmentation and colored by our method.

3.2.2 Diabetic retinopathy type 2

Type 2 diabetic retinopathy was analyzed from 16 DR2 EFP images showing vascular dysfunction. **Table 3** shows the diverse grades of microaneurysms, and hemorrhages, exudates, new vessels, and venous irregularities not appreciated in original DR2 EFP images. This indicates that the proposed method can define a wider DR grading as a future assignment. The oximetric density function shows a deep decay in O_2 in the 200 to 255 Red scale in all images and a new rectifier wave in the lowest SaO_2, which means loss of O_2 transportation by the predominance of venues tree. The SaO_2 metrics show evident differences among all images, which

Table 2.
Application of the pseudo color method applied to patients DR1–1 to DR1–4 (Diabetic Retinopathy Type 1 [13]).
In addition to the graphing of the repetition of the values obtained from the vector of each image.

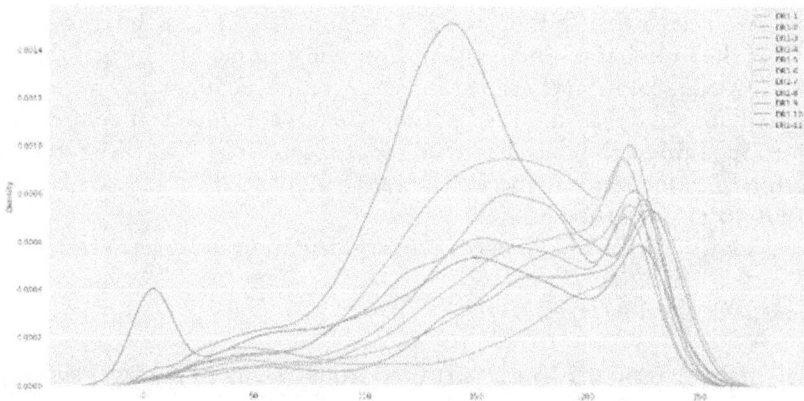

Figure 10.
Shows the comparative performance of the density in the 11 type 1 diabetic retinopathy eyes from SatO$_2$.

let us think we have a new tool for following diabetic patients and comparing their own EFP images through time. The reader must notice an increment in the SaO$_2$. However, this phenomenon is correlated with blood increase, not in the retina

Table 3.
Application of the pseudo color method applied to patients DR2–1 to DR2–4 (Diabetic Retinopathy Type 2 [13]). In addition to the graphing of the repetition of the values obtained from the vector of each image.

microvasculature but in microaneurysms, hemorrhages, and new vessels. Another important issue is the absence of a black background, indicating inflammatory process.

Table 3 shows the diverse grades of microaneurysms, hemorrhages, new vessels, and venous irregularities in DR2 SatO₂ analysis.

3.2.3 Diabetic retinopathy type 3

Results from Diabetic Retinopathy type 3 analysis show a more profound degradation of the microvasculature. **Table 4** shows SaO₂ analysis from 10 EFP images previously classified as DR3. Images are from [13].

The oximetric density function clearly shows decomposition in the waveform in the 200–255 range. The rectifier sinewave that appeared in the healthy eye is no longer there.

Table 4.
*Application of the pseudo color method applied to patients DR3–1 to DR3–4 (Diabetic Retinopathy Type 3 [13]).
In addition to the graphing of the repetition of the values obtained from the vector of each image.*

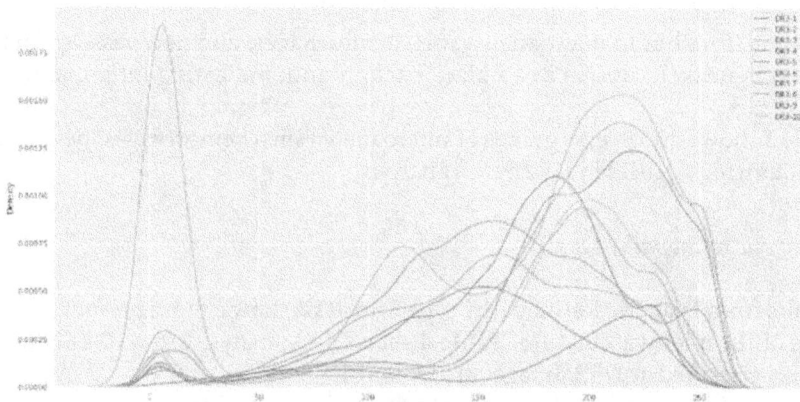

Figure 11.
Shows the comparative performance of the density in the 10 type 3 diabetic retinopathy eyes from SatO₂.

Table 4 shows the varying degrees of microaneurysms, hemorrhages, new vessels, and venous irregularities in the DR3 SatO$_2$ analysis (**Figure 11**).

4. Discussion

Vessel segmentation is an increased research field, and there is no doubt better solutions are coming to differentiate vessels from arteries. However, that differentiation is not only in the image segmentation area or in traditional methods of classifying diabetic retinopathy grading. Our results show that DR in any of their grading shows a wide range of differences that must be reclassified. This will help better follow-up with diabetic patients, observing the illness evolution closely without expecting to detect the transition from DR1 to DR2 or DR3. Assuming that better vessel segmentation results are obtained, the results shown indicate that, if associated with SatO$_2$ vectors, the vessel color images are numerical vectors that can be studied as a mathematical function. This opens new opportunities for researchers and physicians to study DR not only from sight observation but also from deep learning and artificial intelligence tools.

4.1 Healthy eyes: A comparative analysis

Maliheh Miri et al. [7] proposed a method to distinguish arteries from veins in the retina microvasculature in 2017. This work is a significant contribution to the field that seeks an automatic procedure to classify arteries and veins. For comparison with our proposal, the results of the same DRIVE EFP obtained with both the Maliheh Miri method and the proposed method are shown. **Figure 12(A–D)** shows the DRIVE EFP used in both studies.

Figure 13 shows Maliheh Miri et al. [7] results for distinguishing arteries from veins in the retina microvasculature. Blue represents the vein system, and red shows the arterial retina microvasculature. The segmentation algorithm used by Maliheh Miri is based on contrast and illumination differences between arteria and veins. Those differences, as shown, show the arterial and veins with two colors (a,b,c,d); however, they do not identify the SatO$_2$ performance in the microvasculature.

Figure 14 shows the results of the proposed segmentation method of arteries and veins using the same DRIVE EFP images as Maliheh Miri. The segmented

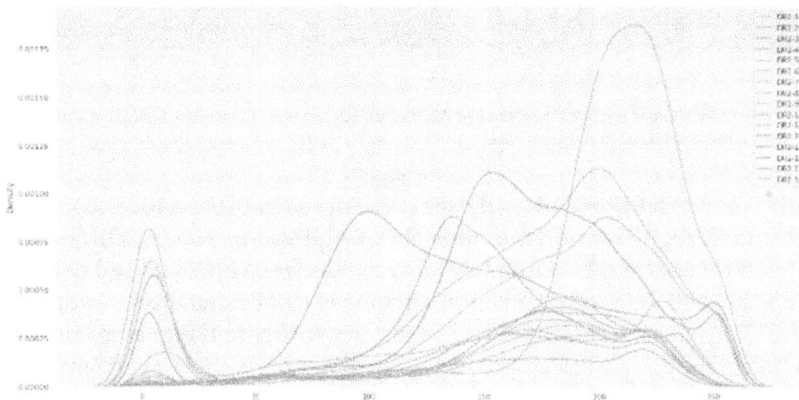

Figure 12.
Shows the comparative performance of the density in the 16 type 2 diabetic retinopathy eyes from SatO$_2$.

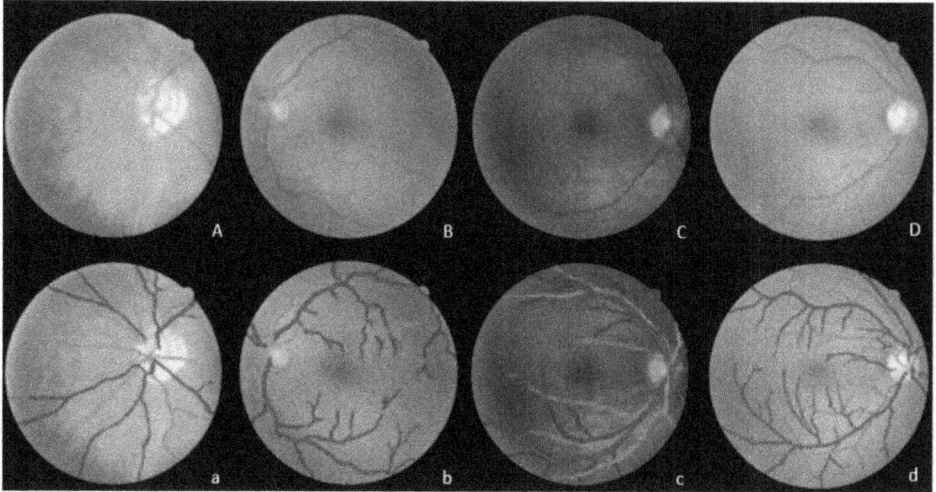

Figure 13.
Maliheh Miri et al. [7] proposed a method to distinguish arteries from veins in the retinal microvasculature. The blue color represents the venous system, the red color shows the arterial microvasculature of the retina. (A, B, C, D) shows the original images extracted from the DRIVE database [11], while (a, b, c, d) shows the segmentation method to identify such microvasculature.

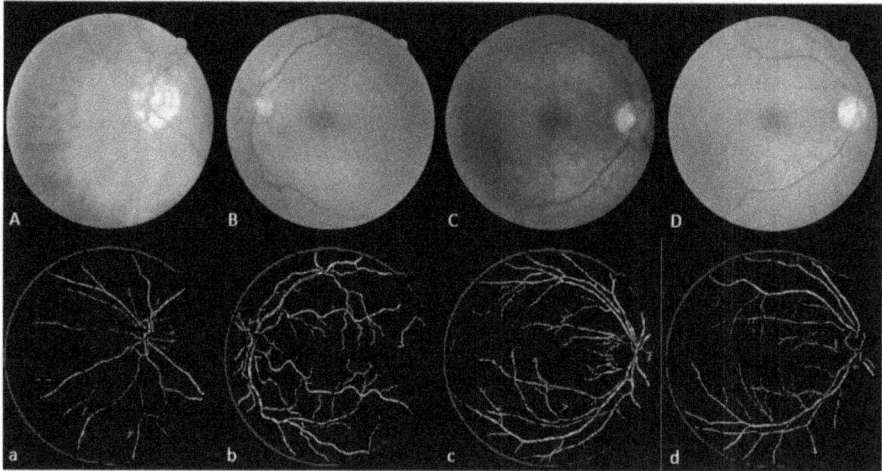

Figure 14.
(A, B, C, D) shows the images reported by Maliheh Miri et al. [7] extracted from the DRIVE database, while (a, b, c, d) shows the application of the oxygen saturation estimation method proposed in this research work.

trajectories found in **Figure 14(a–d)** are the same as in **Figure 10(a–d)**. This means that both segmentation methods obtain equivalent results. Differences in colorimetry were found. Maliheh Miri proposes fixed blue and red colors, as shown in **Figure 13**. The assigned colors in our method reflect the O_2 content in each pixel along the arteries branches' veins, according to the gray levels in the original image for both arteries and veins. Both methods show precise trajectories from the microvasculature supported by a black background. The black background without blood signals is evidence of a healthy eye showing noninflammatory processes.

5. Conclusions and future challenges

The research presents an innovative method to quantify oxygen saturation in the retinal vascular system by analyzing fundus images. This method proposes the Oximetric Distribution Function (ODF), which transforms images into vectors where each pixel of the circulatory system has a specific gray level and an estimate of oxygen saturation. This methodology allows detailed and accurate tracking of oxygen saturation, providing a fundamental graphical tool for understanding retinal vascular function. ODF provides not only a numerical representation but also a graphical visualization of ocular health status, which has both clinical and research applications.

The proposed method significantly improves accuracy and traceability compared to current methods by providing a detailed map of oxygen saturation rather than an average measurement. This may have important implications for the diagnosis and monitoring of oxygen saturation-related eye diseases, such as retinal vascular disease.

The results of the oximetric function vary according to the parameters of the camera used and the errors in the conversion from spherical to flat images. The research highlights the need to adjust fundus imaging technology to minimize errors, such as those associated with the conversion of curved areas to flat images, and to normalize Lambert-Beer's law alpha value. This normalization is crucial to ensure the consistency and reliability of the results obtained by the proposed method.

A significant contribution of this study is the postulation of the hypothesis of quantifiable and visible vascular inflammation in the retina, with preliminary results suggesting the possible detection and measurement of such inflammation. This finding has the potential to significantly improve the diagnosis and monitoring of various ocular diseases. However, to ensure the validity of these results, the analysis requires images obtained from the same fundus camera and captured at the same wavelength, highlighting the importance of uniformity in the image acquisition process.

Future research will focus on the normalization of alpha values and the consideration of errors due to diffraction and light scattering, factors that have not been considered so far but that directly affect the images obtained by fundus cameras. These investigations will contribute to establishing guidelines and standards that allow effective comparison of results between different equipment, providing greater confidence in the clinical interpretation of the oximetry data obtained. Understanding these variabilities and implementing the necessary corrections are essential to ensure the consistency and validity of the results in different clinical contexts.

Acknowledgements

The authors thank CONAHCyT and the National Polytechnic Institute for their financial support throughout the work.

Conflict of interest

The authors declare that they have no conflicts of interest.

Author details

Luis Niño-de-Rivera[1*], Erwin Michel Davila-Iniesta[1] and Félix Gil-Carrasco[2]

1 Artificial Vision Lab, ESIME UC, Instituto Politécnico Nacional, IPN México, México

2 Asociación Para Evitar la Ceguera, APEC México, Mexico

*Address all correspondence to: luisninoderivera@gmail.com

IntechOpen

References

[1] Tan T-E, Wong TY. Diabetic retinopathy: Looking forward to 2030. Frontiers in Endocrinology. 2023;**13**:1077669. DOI: 10.3389/fendo.2022.1077669

[2] Yang Z, Tan T-E, Shao Y, Wong TY, Li XR. Classification of diabetic retinopathy: Past, present and future. Frontiers in Endocrinology. 2022;**13**:1079217. DOI: 10.3389/fendo.2022.1079217

[3] Davila-Iniesta E-M, Niño-de-Rivera L. A New Method to Manipulate Conventional OCT Images to Measure Changes in the Relative Haemoglobin Oxygen Saturation. London, UK: IntechOpen; 2023. DOI: 10.5772/intechopen.110884

[4] Stefánsson E, Olafsdottir OB, Eliasdottir TS, Vehmeijer W, Einarsdottir AB, Bek T, et al. Retinal oximetry: Metabolic imaging for diseases of the retina and brain. Progress in Retinal and Eye Research. 2019;**70**:1-22. DOI: 10.1016/j.preteyeres.2019.04.001. ISSN 1350-9462

[5] Davila-Iniesta E, Guerrero-Gonzalez S, Santiago-Amaya J, Castillo-Juarez P, Niño-de-Rivera-Oyarzabal L. False color method for retinal oximetry. Journal of Biomedical Science and Engineering. 2019;**12**:533-544. DOI: 10.4236/jbise.2019.1212044

[6] Kumar JRH, Seelamantula CS, Mohan A, Shetty R, Berendschot TJM, Webers CAB. Automatic analysis of normative retinal oximetry images. PLoS One. 2020;**15**(5):e0231677. DOI: 10.1371/journal.pone.0231677

[7] Malihe M, Zahra A, Hossein R, Raheleh K. A comprehensive study of retinal vessel classification methods in fundus images. Journal of Medical Signals and Sensors. 2017;7(2):59-70

[8] Hirsch K, Cubbidge RP, Heitmar R. Dual wavelength retinal vessel oximetry – Influence of fundus pigmentation. Eye. 2023;**37**:2246-2251. DOI: 10.1038/s41433-022-02325-7

[9] Karlsson RA, Olafsdottir OB, Helgadottir V, Belhadj S, Eliasdottir TS, Stefansson E, et al. Automation improves repeatability of retinal oximetry measurements. PLoS One. 2021;**16**(12):e0260120. DOI: 10.1371/journal.pone.0260120

[10] Kristjansdottir JV, Hardarson SH, Harvey AR, Olafsdottir OB, Eliasdottir TS, Stefánsson E. Choroidal oximetry with a noninvasive spectrophotometric oximeter. Investigative Ophthalmology & Visual Science. 2013;**54**(5):3234-3239

[11] Eliasdottir TS. Retinal oximetry and systemic arterial oxygen levels. Acta Ophthalmologica. 2018;**96, thesis 113**:1-44

[12] Budai A, Bock R, Maier A, Hornegger J, Michelson G. Robust vessel segmentation in fundus images. International Journal of Biomedical Imaging. 2013;**2013**:154860. DOI: 10.1155/2013/154860. Epub 2013 Dec 12

[13] Cen L-P, Ji J, Lin JW, Si Tong J, Lin H, Li TP, et al. Automatic detection of 39 fundus diseases and conditions in retinal photographs using deep neural networks. Nature Communications. 2021;**12**(1):4828. DOI: 10.1038/s41467-021-25138-w

[14] Oakley N, Hill DW, Joplin GF, Kohner EM, Fraser TR, Diabetic retinopathy. I. The assessment of severity and progress by comparison with a set of standard fundus photographs. Diabetologia. 1967;**3**(4):402-405. DOI: 10.1007/BF02342633

Chapter 6

Methyl Alcohol Intoxication: Recognition and Management with Arterial Blood Gases

Canan Akman, Neslihan Ergün Süzer and Özgür Karcıoğlu

Abstract

Intoxication with methanol and other toxic alcohols remains a major public health issue in most parts of the world. Recognition of pathological mechanisms and outcomes that can be encountered following methanol intake is necessary for all healthcare providers. Symptoms begin as early as half an hour and if there is no treatment, progress to decompensate metabolic acidosis within 12 hours. Seizures, acidosis, hypoglycemia, and blindness often complicate the picture. Acute kidney injury requires emergency hemodialysis. General and fundoscopic examination, biochemistry, and arterial blood gas analysis comprise the main diagnostic arsenal. Intravenous sodium bicarbonate, correction of electrolyte imbalance, ethanol, folate/leucovorin, and hemodialysis are crucial agents for effective treatment in selected patients with specific indications. The basic steps in the management are initiated in the prehospital area, emergency department, and intensive care unit and should be closely monitored for the prevention of long-term sequelae. This chapter is intended to summarize the clinical presentation and emergency management of these cases within the framework of basic physiological and biochemical events that follow toxic alcohol consumption including methanol.

Keywords: methanol, methyl alcohol intoxication, toxic alcohol, poisoning, hemodialysis, arterial blood gases

1. Introduction

Methanol or methyl alcohol is a type of toxic alcohol that can cause death by leading to severe poisoning just after consumption. The compound is obtained by distillation from charcoal and was first used in ancient Egypt for mummification [1]. Due to the solvent effect, it can be sold legally because it is widely used in certain industries including dry cleaning, automotive, and energy. As a colorless, odorless substance, methyl alcohol is usually not distinguished from ethyl alcohol when ingested orally. Therefore, it can be used especially in the illegal production of alcoholic beverages because its cost is lower than ethyl alcohol. Methyl alcohol poisoning (MAP) is increasingly common in emergency departments (ED) due to widespread consumption of illegally produced beverages in recent years. Rarely, there are accidental oral intakes of eau de cologne, spirits, disinfectant agents, industrial alcohol, etc., resulting in significant clinical conditions and MAP. It has been reported that it can also cause poisoning by inhalation or dermal route, mostly accidentally.

Lifesaving steps in patients with MAP include early referral of patients to the ED or hospital, early diagnosis and effective antidote treatment, as well as the initiation of hemodialysis in the necessary patients. Provided that the level of methyl alcohol cannot be measured in most institutions, difficulty in the recognition and management of MAP can be overcome by the increased awareness of society and by knowing the early clinical diagnostic findings, especially about MAP by physicians.

2. Physicochemical properties and mechanism of action

Methyl alcohol is a liposoluble compound that can be absorbed orally, through inhalation or through the skin. Severe cases of intoxication reported by exposure from different routes are available [2, 3]. When methyl alcohol is taken orally, it is absorbed very quickly from the gastric mucosa and reaches the plasma peak concentration in about 30–60 minutes [4]. Methanol is a water-soluble compound unbound to protein weighing 32 Daltons. The volume of distribution (Vd) is 0.6 L/kg and the endogenous clearance is 0.7 mL/kg/min [5, 6].

Dose-response relation: Intake of a small amount—even 8–10 mL—of methanol can cause serious toxicity. About 25–30 mL can result in MAP leading to permanent blindness, while 1 mL/kg or 100 ml of methanol intake can cause death of the patient. Methyl alcohol is converted into formaldehyde by enzymatic reaction with alcohol dehydrogenase (AlcoDH). Formaldehyde is metabolized by aldehyde dehydrogenase (AldeDH) to formic acid [7]. Formic acid is converted into CO_2 and water by using folic acid as cofactor and thus completes the metabolism of methanol.

Clinical signs and symptoms associated with MAP can begin as short as 40 minutes, depending on the type and amount of exposure, while it may extend up to 72 hours after ingestion taken with ethanol (antidote) [8].

Usually, the period between ingestion and the appearance of signs and symptoms is the time taken for methanol to turn into toxic metabolites. The metabolism of methyl alcohol through AlcoDH and AldeDH leads to the formation of metabolites that contribute to the increased anion gap. Therefore, the clinical course of MAP in these patients is manifested by high anion gap metabolic acidosis (HAGMA). Formic acid, the metabolite of methanol, is toxic to many tissues. Formic acid causes cytochrome C oxidase inhibition in the electron transport chain, leading to cellular dysfunction and destructive organ damage. Formic acid also inhibits oxidative phosphorylation, leading to augmented anaerobic metabolism increasing lactate. This also contributes to metabolic acidosis in those with MAP.

3. Diagnostic tests

The first critical step to establish a diagnosis is to suspect intoxication in MAP, as in all patients presented with poisoning. Along with clinical suspicion, adjunctive diagnostic tests are important for definitive diagnosis and management. Fingertip blood glucose measurement, complete blood count, blood biochemistry, drug levels such as paracetamol and salicylate, electrocardiography (ECG), pregnancy test (B-HCG) for all female patients of childbearing age, should be performed on all patients who present with significant signs and/or symptoms of poisoning. Arterial or venous blood gases and electrolytes (to determine the anion gap), kidney function tests, lactate level, complete urinalysis, and serum osmolarity should be ordered in association with testing for ethanol, methanol, and other toxic alcohol levels in patients with suspected poisoning with methanol or other toxic alcohol.

The best method for the definitive diagnosis of MAP is the measurement of methanol levels in the blood. Levels above 20 mg/dL are toxic, while >50 mg/dL causes severe central nervous system toxicity and around 200 mg/dL is lethal [6]. However, the level of methanol in the blood is not available in most EDs. In recent years, several studies have recommended bedside tests that can measure formic acid levels, but their use is still limited [9, 10]. The normal level of methanol measured in the blood does not exclude MAP, because the blood level of methanol is reduced as a function of time. Therefore, the laboratory should be supported with current clinical findings for diagnosis.

Patients with MAP have a HAGMA due to the metabolism of methanol to organic acids, both the osmolar gap and the anion deficit are increased [11, 12]. If metabolic acidosis in ED patients cannot be clearly explained, poisoning should be considered first, and MAP should be a priority among the presumptive diagnoses.

Osmolality vs. osmolarity: Direct measurements (i.e., measurements reported from an osmometer) measure osmolality (mosm/kg water) while calculated measurements, as described below, are estimates of osmolarity (mosm/L solution) [13]. In routine clinical practice, these two measurements are virtually the same and are often used interchangeably.

Osmolar gap is the difference between measured and calculated serum osmolarity. If the amount of alcohol ingested is known, the osmolar gap can be calculated exactly.

On the other hand, osmolality is a measurement of the number of moles of dissolved particles per kg of solvent (for clinical purposes, water is the solvent). Levels of serum osmolal gap can be used as a valuable instrument in the suspicion of intoxication with various alcohol types. Normally osmolal gap are expected to be lower than 10 mOsm/kg). Osmolal gap higher than 20 mOsm/kg mostly follows ingestion of toxic alcohols (i.e., methanol, ethylene glycol, isopropanol, propylene glycol, diethylene glycol), or organic solvents (acetone) but rarely of ethanol alone. Some reports identified an increase in the osmolal gap may be a result of ethanol intoxication solely [14].

$$\text{Osmolarity}\left(\text{Normal}\,285 \pm 10\,\text{mOsm}/\text{L}\right) = \left(2\text{xNa}\right) + \text{Glu}/18 + \text{BUN}/2,8 + \text{Methanol}/3,2 \quad (1)$$

$$\text{Calculated osmolarity} = \left(2\text{xNa}\right) + \text{Glu}/18 + \text{BUN}/2,8 \quad (2)$$

$$\text{Osmolar gap}\left(\text{normal}\,0-5\right) = \text{Measured} - \text{Calculated} \quad (3)$$

$$\text{Anion gap}\left(\text{Normal}\,8 \pm 4\right) = \text{Na} + - \left(\text{HCO3} - + \text{Cl} -\right) \quad (4)$$

Formic acid inhibits oxidative phosphorylation, leading to increased anaerobic metabolism, which causes hyperlactatemia in patients with MAP. Lactate levels will also be high in patients with hypotension (leading to hypoperfusion) and end-organ failure.

Basal ganglia necrosis can be seen in the patients exposed to methanol and is manifested by bleeding and edema in computed tomography (CT) and magnetic resonance imaging (MRI) [15, 16]. These imaging methods must be ordered in patients with altered mental status or other neurological deficits.

4. Differential diagnosis

There are several clinical conditions that cause HAGMA, including hyperlactatemia, status epilepticus, shock states, mesenteric ischemia, diabetic ketoacidosis, metformin overdose (**Table 1**). Intoxications with agents including metformin, aspirin, other toxic alcohols, and aluminum phosphide should also be considered in the differential diagnosis in patients with metabolic acidosis.

Laboratory findings: MAP can be distinguished from isopropyl alcohol poisoning by the fact that isopropyl alcohol is metabolized into ketone instead of acidic compounds. Therefore, osmolar gap and ketosis are apparent without acidosis. Ethylene glycol toxicity, on the other hand, causes HAGMA associated with increased osmolar gap.

On the other hand, recent studies emphasize that the measurement of blood formate concentrations is required for immediate management and investigation of the cause of death [15]. The authors indicated that headspace gas chromatography–mass spectrometry (HS-GC-MS) and a formate assay kit are valuable adjuncts in the diagnosis of MAP.

Bedside testing of formate can help in establishing the diagnosis of MAP. Detection of formate with the enzyme formate oxidase (FOX) is a viable alternative to diagnose MAP simple and fast. The sensitivity of the FOX-enzyme was 100% and the specificity was 97% while no false positives were detected [16].

5. Clinical findings

Although the signs of poisoning are often specific in the late period of MAP, most of the early findings are nonspecific. Early signs involving the gastrointestinal tract such as nausea, vomiting, and abdominal pain are prominent. Patients often have signs of drunkenness following ingestion of alcohol, which renders history-taking quite difficult. Clinical manifestations of MAP are characterized by different findings in three periods. Complaints that begin with nonspecific gastrointestinal findings in the first stage, wane

M	Methanol, Metformin
U	Uremia
D	Diabetic ketoacidosis
P	Paraldehyde
I	Isoniazide, Iron
L	Lactate
E	Ethylene glycol
S	Salicylate

Table 1.
Mnemonic of causes of high anion gap metabolic acidosis: `MUD PILES`.

Clinical stages	Signs and symptoms
Stage 1 (the first hours after intake)	• drunkenness
	• Gastrointestinal system irritation
	• Increased osmolar gap
Stage 2 (latent stage; 3 to 30 hours)	Signs and symptoms may be subtle or absent
Stage 3	• Visual impairments or blindness
	• High anion gap metabolic acidosis
	• Abdominal pain, vomiting, pancreatitis
	• Altered mental status, seizures, coma
	• Kidney injury
	• Myocardial dysfunction
	• Cerebral hemorrhage

Table 2.
Clinical staging in methanol poisoning.

in the second stage and become quite similar to symptoms after classical alcohol intake for a short period (Latent Period). This period may last for 2 hours, or extend up to 1 or 2 days, especially if the patient had ingested ethyl alcohol concurrently.

Blurred vision, double vision, photophobia, and early or late blindness may occur after the latent period, accompanied by metabolic acidosis [17, 18]. The severity of acidosis at the time of admission may be associated with the degree of persistent visual impairment; however, more studies are needed to assess this relationship. The level of consciousness may vary from patient to patient. Findings of clinical staging in methanol poisoning are given in **Table 2**.

6. Metabolic status

Increased anion gap ensues with metabolic acidosis with the metabolism of methanol in the body. The investigation of venous blood gases is essential in the diagnosis of MAP to detect the presence of metabolic acidosis in patients with alcohol intake. In patients with nonspecific clinical manifestations of alcohol intake, especially in the first and second stages, the presence of osmolar gap with calculated blood osmolarity is critical in the diagnosis of MAP in institutions where anion gap and blood osmolarity can be measured. While osmolar gap is more predictive and valuable in the early stages of MAP, it begins to decrease and the anion gap becomes even more important in diagnosis with the accumulation of metabolites.

7. Ocular findings

Untreated MAP causes injury to the optic nerve and retinal epithelial cells, leading to symmetric or asymmetric blurred vision or blindness in severe poisoning. These findings result from the effects of methanol metabolites and formic acid, which may be subtle or absent until 48–72 hours. On ophthalmological examination, central scotoma, hyperemia, paleness in the optic disc, and papillary edema are characteristically detected. It is unclear why the eyes are affected by MAP, while some other tissues are spared, which attracts the attention of ongoing research [19–21]. MAP can cause non-reversible toxic optic neuropathy. Acidemia associated with HAGMA and a suspicious fundus ophthalmic examination allows a fast diagnosis [22].

8. Neurological findings

Depending on the amount taken, all alcohols cause a change in the level of consciousness and intoxication. However, alcohol tolerance is usually developed in chronic alcoholics, and signs of intoxication can be seen even when the patient's level of consciousness is normal. Neurological signs of MAP occur with increased levels of presynaptic gamma-aminobutyric acid (GABA) receptors, N Methyl-D-aspartic acid (NMDA) inhibition of glutamate receptors, and GABA. Patients with MAP may experience headaches, central nervous system depression, coma, and seizures [23, 24]. Imaging is definitely recommended in patients with a change of consciousness or neurological deficits, which may predict putaminal necrosis, and/or intracranial hemorrhage (e.g., subarachnoid hemorrhage, putaminal intraparenchymal bleeding).

9. Imaging

Lesions in the basal ganglia, abnormal appearance in the caudate nuclei and necrosis in the putamen with or without bleeding can be detected in computed tomography and magnetic resonance imaging, especially in patients with neurological deficits [25, 26]. The appearance of these lesions is associated with grave outcomes, while eye-related complications and cerebral lesions may form permanent sequelae [27].

10. Treatment

MAP can cause coma and cardiorespiratory compromise, which prompt immediate evaluation of ABC and fingertip glucose measurement, along with the stabilization of vital signs and resuscitation of the patients. The management comprises IV sodium bicarbonate, correction of electrolyte imbalance, ethyl alcohol, folate, and hemodialysis, if necessary [28]. The basic steps in the approach must be undertaken in the ED and followed up with meticulous monitoring in the ICU for salvage as well as prevention of long-term sequelae.

Control of the airway patency through tracheal intubation may be required. The cause of hypotension, which is common in these patients, is initially secondary to vomiting, fluid loss, and vasodilation, whereas severe metabolic acidosis and multiple organ failure are prominent in the later phases. Adequate replacement of crystalloid fluids and inotropic drugs are administered in the treatment of these severe conditions. Since methanol is absorbed very quickly from the gastrointestinal tract, using gastric lavage and activated charcoal is not indicated [29]. In addition to supportive treatment, antidote treatment, and hemodialysis are among the most critical steps to save lives.

11. Antidotes

Indications for the administration of antidotes are determined by clinical and laboratory findings in a patient considered to have MAP. A history of methanol

Criteria
1. The serum methanol level is above 6.2 mmol/L or 20 mg/dL
2. Osmolar gap is >10 mOsm/L with a history compatible with a toxic dose of methanol intake
3. Having at least two of the following conditions with a history of suspected methanol intake • Arterial pH <7,3 • Bicarbonate <20 mmol/L • Osmolar gap >10 mOsm/L • High anion gap metabolic acidosis with compatible clinical manifestations

Table 3.
Indications for antidote treatment in methanol poisoning.

intake, unexplained HAGMA or osmolar gap with another possible cause necessitate antidote treatment. The elimination half-life of methanol is between 2 and 14 hours in the absence of antidote therapy. ADH inhibition with fomepizole or any other agent can extend the elimination half-life of methanol to an average of 54 hours. Indications of antidote treatment are given in **Table 3** [30].

12. Fomepizole

Fomepizole is a competitive antagonist for the ADH enzyme and an effective antidote used for MAP. After an IV loading dose of 15 mg/kg, 10 mg/kg IV, the agent is repeated in 12 hours, up to 4 doses in total. Fomepizole treatment has many advantages over ethanol and needs to be administered every 12 hours to provide stronger ADH inhibition than ethanol. Its effect lasts longer and eliminates the need for ethanol infusion. There will be no significant difference in serum concentration when given IV or PO. Due to its effectiveness and lower adverse effect profile compared to ethanol, fomepizole may reduce the need for admissions to intensive care in selected patients. There are some published data from centers where methyl alcohol level can be measured urgently in patients who present early, in whom fomepizole application can eliminate the need for hemodialysis, but these conditions are not possible in most circumstances [30]. In patients receiving hemodialysis, two different regimens are recommended for fomepizole. In the alternative regimen, the loading dose remains the same, but the second dose is recommended to be administered at 12 hours instead of 6 hours. Additional doses may be repeated every 4 hours or at a rate of 1–1.5 mg/kg/h after loading dose, and continuous infusion may also be administered during hemodialysis [6]. The drawbacks comprise the need for transportation, high cost, and unavailability of the drug except for poisoning centers [31]. Fomepizole administration may cause bradycardia and hypotension, thus patients should be monitored during administration [32].

13. Ethyl alcohol

Ethanol and fomepizole are strong inhibitors of ADH. If fomepizole is not available and the administration of hemodialysis in patients will be delayed, an IV loading dose of 10%' ethanol, 10 mL/kg/h, followed by an infusion of 1 mL/kg/h to maintain a serum concentration about 150 mg/dL can be given as a competitive ADH substrate.

Respiratory depression, hypotension, flushing, hypoglycemia, and gastrointestinal symptoms may develop during the treatment. Patients treated with IV ethanol will generally necessitate follow-up in the ICU. In cases where monitoring is not feasible, ethanol can be administered orally or via a nasogastric tube. When administered orally, 5 mL/kg 20% solution of ethanol will be loaded and repeated at doses of 0.5 mL/kg/h. Ethanol levels must be measured every 1–2 hours in those with ethanol administration [33, 34].

14. Sodium bicarbonate

In patients suspected of MAP, sodium bicarbonate (NaHCO₃) is usually recommended only pH is below 7.3 and NaHCO3 < 20 mEq/L [35]. The goal of this treatment is to mitigate the end-organ damage of acid degradation products, increasing renal excretion, and achievement of a blood pH target (above 7,30). Although there is no consensus on dosage, administration of 1–2 mEq/kg IV is recommended [36].

15. Folic acid and leucovorin

A total of 1 mg/kg (up to 50 mg) of folic acid and leucovorin may be administered IV every 4 hours in those with MAP. The aim is to augment the metabolism of formic acid. Formic acid needs folic acid in the breakdown process as a cofactor. Although the effectiveness of this treatment has been demonstrated in animal experiments, there are ongoing human studies [7].

16. Corticosteroids

There is scarce data on the use of corticosteroids in patients with retinal injury due to MAP, in whom the treatment partially improves ocular symptoms or stops their progression. In a case series with MAP an improvement in vision was observed in most patients receiving corticosteroid therapy [37]. The authors reported that 500 mg methylprednisolone IV every 12 hours, followed by 5 mg/kg prednisolone for up to 2 days, and after 2 weeks may improve eye findings [38, 39].

17. Hemodialysis

Hemodialysis is the recommended method of extracorporeal therapy in MAP, based on the pharmacokinetic properties of methanol and formic acid. Hemodialysis removes methanol and its toxic metabolites from the blood, which institutes acid-base balance. The main indications of the use of hemodialysis are given in **Table 4**. In situations to prevent the formation of formate, ethanol or fomepizole therapy has been quickly initiated, and if there are no acute clinical signs, ECTR does not need to be initiated immediately [40].

Each patient with MAP presented with impaired vision and *de novo* emergence of organ failure is recommended to undergo hemodialysis of MAP without wasting time. Many patients may require recurrent hemodialysis. In cases where hemodialysis cannot be performed due to a patient's hemodynamics or unavailability, continuous renal

1. Hemodialysis indications	a. Coma
	b. Seizures
	c. *De novo* visual impairment
	d. Blood pH <7,15
	e. Persistent acidosis despite supportive treatment and antidotes
	f. Anion gap >24 mmol/L
	g. Methanol level > 700 mg/L (21,8 mmol/L) after fomepizole treatment
	h. Methanol level > 600 mg/L (18,7 mmol/L) after ethanol treatment
	i. Methanol level > 500 mg/L (15,6 mmol/L) if ADH inhibitor (fomepizole) is unavailable
	j. Osmolar gap is informative when methanol levels are not measured
	k. Impaired kidney functions
2. Stopping hemodialysis	a. Methanol level < 200 mg/L (6,2 mmol/L) accompanied by clinical improvement
3. Extracorporeal treatments	a. Intermittent hemodialysis is preferred
	b. Continuous renal replacement therapy or similar methods can be employed when intermittent hemodialysis is not feasible.

Table 4.
Extracorporeal treatment recommendations in patients with methanol poisoning.

replacement therapy is a viable alternative method of venovenous hemodiafiltration, albeit hemodialysis is more effective in removing drugs from the blood than the latter. Hemodialysis treatment can be terminated when the methanol concentration drops below <200 mg/L (6.2 mmol/L) or when clinical relief is observed (improvement of acidosis in blood gas). If possible, dialysis without heparin should be performed, since anticoagulation may worsen hemorrhage. In severe toxicity associated with altered mental status, it should be considered that there may be putaminal necrosis and/or hemorrhage, intracranial hemorrhage, SAH, and massive brain edema.

18. Other treatments

Thiamine (100 mg IV) and Pyridoxine (50 mg IV) may be employed in chronic alcoholics. The antiretroviral drug Abacavir is also a substrate for ADH and slows the metabolism of methanol. It has been recommended in treatment in cases not receiving fomepizole [40]. In addition, neuroprotective effect of erythropoietin against hypoxic damage has been demonstrated in animal experiments. Studies on its use to treat ocular symptoms show promise [41].

19. Outcome and disposition

Although early diagnosis and aggressive treatment are lifesaving, MAP can be highly mortal even after proper treatment. Vision loss and neurodeficits may remain as important sequelae in severe cases. Every patient with suspicion of methanol intake should be kept under follow-up in the ED or ward for around 24 hours to monitor osmolar gap, anionic gap, and blood gases and evaluated clinically for MAP. Occasionally, patients may experience delayed emergence of the classical signs of MAP, especially if they have concurrent ethanol consumption. In EDs, where the follow-up period is shorter due to high patient numbers, the patient(s) must be informed of signs of poisoning while being discharged.

Author details

Canan Akman[1], Neslihan Ergün Süzer[2] and Özgür Karcıoğlu[3*]

1 Department of Emergency Medicine, Canakkale Onsekiz Mart University, Canakkale, Turkey

2 Department of Emergency Medicine, Darica Farabi Education and Research Hospital, Kocaeli, Turkey

3 Department of Emergency Medicine, Istanbul Education and Research Hospital, University of Health Sciences, Istanbul, Turkey

*Address all correspondence to: okarcioglu@gmail.com

IntechOpen

References

[1] Ott J, Gronemann V, Pontzen F, et al. Methanol. In: Ullmann's Encyclopedia of Industrial Chemistry. Weinheim, Germany: Wiley-VCH Verlag GmbH & Co. KGaA; 2012. pp. 1-27. DOI: 10.1002/14356007.a16_465.pub3

[2] Gómez Perera S, Rodríguez Talavera I, Tapia Quijada HE, et al. Secondary visual loss due to inhalation and cutaneous poisoning by methanol and toluene. Presentation of a clinical case. Archivos de la Sociedad Espanola de Oftalmologia. 2020;**95**(5):231-235. DOI: 10.1016/J. OFTAL.2020.02.004

[3] Robledo C, Saracho R. Methanol poisoning by solvent inhalation. Nefrología. 2018;**38**(6):679-680. DOI: 10.1016/J.NEFRO.2018.03.005

[4] Pohanka M. Toxicology and the biological role of methanol and ethanol: Current view. Biomedical papers of the Medical Faculty of the University Palacky, Olomouc, Czechoslovakia. 2016;**160**(1):54-63. DOI: 10.5507/BP.2015.023

[5] Vale A. Methanol. Medicine. 2007;**35**(12):633-634. DOI: 10.1016/J. MPMED.2007.09.014

[6] Mégarbane B. Treatment of patients with ethylene glycol or methanol poisoning: Focus on fomepizole. Open Access Emergency Medicine. 2010;**2**:67. DOI: 10.2147/ OAEM.S5346

[7] Liesivuori J, Savolainen AH. Methanol and formic acid toxicity: Biochemical mechanisms. Pharmacology and Toxicology. 1991;**69**(3):157-163. DOI: 10.1111/J.1600-0773.1991.TB01290.X

[8] Kruse JA. Methanol and ethylene glycol intoxication. Critical Care Clinics. 2012;**28**(4):661-711. DOI: 10.1016/J. CCC.2012.07.002

[9] Hovda KE, Gadeholt G, Evtodienko V, et al. A novel bedside diagnostic test for methanol poisoning using dry chemistry for formate. Scandinavian Journal of Clinical and Laboratory Investigation. 2015;**75**(7):610-614. DOI: 10.3109/00365513.2015.1066847

[10] Hovda KE, Lao YE, Gadeholt G, et al. Formate test for bedside diagnosis of methanol poisoning. Basic and Clinical Pharmacology and Toxicology. 2021;**129**(1):86-88. DOI: 10.1111/ BCPT.13597

[11] Kraut JA, Kurtz I. Toxic alcohol ingestions: Clinical features, diagnosis, and management. Clinical Journal of the American Society of Nephrology. 2008;**3**(1):208-225. DOI: 10.2215/ CJN.03220807

[12] Gallagher N, Edwards FJ. The diagnosis and management of toxic alcohol poisoning in the emergency department: A review article. Advanced Journal of Emergency Medicine. 2019;**3**(3):28. DOI: 10.22114/AJEM. V0I0.153

[13] Emmett M, Palmer BF. Serum Osmolal Gap. The Netherlands; 24 Oct 2024. Available from: https:// www. uptodate.com/contents/serum-osmolal-gap [Accessed: February 27, 2025]

[14] Liontos A, Samanidou V, Athanasiou L, Filippas-Ntekouan S, Milionis C. Acute ethanol intoxication: An overlooked cause of high anion gap metabolic acidosis with a marked increase in serum osmolal gap. Cureus. 2023;**15**(4):e37292. DOI: 10.7759/ cureus.37292

[15] Yoshida H, Harada K, Sakamoto Y, Yoshimura J, Shimazu T, Matsumoto H. Comparison of quantitative values of headspace gas chromatography--mass spectrometry and a formate quantification kit in blood formate quantification. Journal of Analytical Toxicology. 2023;**47**(4):338-345. DOI: 10.1093/jat/bkac107

[16] Lao YE, Heyerdahl F, Jacobsen D, Hovda KE. An enzymatic assay with formate oxidase for point-of-care diagnosis of methanol g. Basic & Clinical Pharmacology & Toxicology. 2022;**131**(6):547-554. DOI: 10.1111/bcpt.13789. Epub 2022 Sep 17

[17] Paasma R, Hovda KE, Hassanian-Moghaddam H, et al. Risk factors related to poor outcome after methanol poisoning and the relation between outcome and antidotes – A multicenter study. Clinical Toxicology. 2012;**50**(9):823-831. DOI: 10.3109/15563650.2012.728224

[18] McMahon DM, Winstead S, Weant KA. Toxic alcohol ingestions: Focus on ethylene glycol and methanol. Advanced Emergency Nursing Journal. 2009;**31**(3):206-213. DOI: 10.1097/TME.0b013e3181ad8be8

[19] Newman N, Biousse V. Diagnostic approach to vision loss. Continuum (Minneap Minn). 2014;**20**(4 Neuro-Ophthalmology):785-815. DOI: 10.1212/01.CON.0000453317.67637.46

[20] Chung TN, Kim SW, Park YS, et al. Unilateral blindness with third cranial nerve palsy and abnormal enhancement of extraocular muscles on magnetic resonance imaging of orbit after the ingestion of methanol. Emergency Medicine Journal. 2010;**27**(5):409-410. DOI: 10.1136/EMJ.2009.084277

[21] Treichel JL, Murray TG, Lewandowski MF, et al. Retinal toxicity in methanol poisoning. Retina. 2004;**24**(2):309-312. DOI: 10.1097/00006982-200404000-00023

[22] Figuerola B, Mendoza A, Roca M, Lacorzana J. Severe visual loss by inhalation of methanol. Romanian Journal of Ophthalmology. 2021;**65**(2):176-179. DOI: 10.22336/rjo.2021.34

[23] Ariwodola OJ, Weiner JL. Ethanol potentiation of GABAergic synaptic transmission may be self-limiting: Role of presynaptic GABA(B) receptors. The Journal of Neuroscience. 2004;**24**(47):10679-10686. DOI: 10.1523/JNEUROSCI.1768-04.2004

[24] Symington L, Jackson L, Klaassen B. Toxic alcohol but not intoxicated - A case report. Scottish Medical Journal. 2005;**50**(3):129-130. DOI: 10.1177/003693300505000314

[25] Aisa TM, Ballut OM. Methanol intoxication with cerebral hemorrhage. Neurosciences (Riyadh). 2016;**21**(3):275-277. DOI: 10.17712/nsj.2016.3.20150592

[26] Jain N, Himanshu D, Verma SP, et al. Methanol poisoning: Characteristic MRI findings. Annals of Saudi Medicine. 2013;**33**(1):68-69. DOI: 10.5144/0256-4947.2012.26.5.1114

[27] McLean DR, Jacobs H, Mielke BW. Methanol poisoning: A clinical and pathological study. Annals of Neurology. 1980;**8**(2):161-167. DOI: 10.1002/ANA.410080206

[28] Kadam DB, Salvi S, Chandanwale A. Methanol poisoning. Journal of Association of Physicians of India. 2018;**66**(4):47-50

[29] Elwell RJ, Darouian P, Bailie GR, et al. Delayed absorption and post-dialysis rebound in a case of acute methanol poisoning. The American

Journal of Emergency Medicine. 2004;**22**(2):126-127. DOI: 10.1016/J. AJEM.2003.12.017

[30] Hovda KE, Jacobsen D. Expert opinion: Fomepizole may ameliorate the need for hemodialysis in methanol poisoning. Human and Experimental Toxicology. 2008;**27**(7):539-546. DOI: 10.1177/0960327108095992

[31] Brent J, McMartin K, Phillips S, et al. Fomepizole for the treatment of methanol poisoning. The New England Journal of Medicine. 2001;**344**(6):424-429. DOI: 10.1056/ NEJM200102083440605

[32] Lepik KJ, Brubacher JR, DeWitt CR, et al. Bradycardia and hypotension associated with fomepizole infusion during hemodialysis. Clinical Toxicology. 2008;**46**(6):570-573. DOI: 10.1080/15563650701725128

[33] Sivilotti MLA. Methanol and Ethylene Glycol Poisoning: Management. The Netherlands: UpToDate; 26 Feb 2024. Available from: https://www. uptodate.com/contents/methanol- and-ethylene-glycol-poisoning- management?search=methanol%20 poisoning&source=search_ res ult&selectedTitle=2~40&us age_ type=default&display_ rank=2#H4284666786 [Accessed: February 10, 2022]

[34] Elenhorn JM, Schonwald S, Ordog G, et al. Ellenhorn's Medical Toxicology: Diagnosis and Treatment of Human Poisoning. 2nd ed. Baltimore, MD: Williams and Wilkins; 1997. p. 2047. ISBN 0-683-30031-8

[35] Naraqi S, Dethlefs RF, Slobodniuk RA, et al. An outbreak of acute methyl alcohol intoxication. Australian and New Zealand Journal of Medicine. 1979;**9**(1):65-68. DOI: 10.1111/ J.1445-5994.1979.TB04116.X

[36] Barceloux DG, Krenzelok EP, Olson K, et al. American academy of clinical toxicology practice guidelines on the treatment of ethylene glycol poisoning. Ad hoc committee. Journal of Toxicology. Clinical Toxicology. 1999;**37**(5):537. DOI: 10.1081/ CLT-100102445

[37] Shukla M, Shikoh I, Saleem A. Intravenous methylprednisolone could salvage vision in methyl alcohol poisoning. Indian Journal of Ophthalmology. 2006;**54**(1):68-69. DOI: 10.4103/0301-4738.21628

[38] Sodhi PK, Goyal JL, Mehta Ms DK. Methanol-induced optic neuropathy: Treatment with intravenous high dose steroids. International Journal of Clinical Practice. 2001;**55**(9):599-602

[39] Sanaei-Zadeh H. What are the therapeutic effects of high-dose intravenous prednisolone in methanol- induced toxic optic neuropathy? Journal of Ocular Pharmacology and Therapeutics. 2012;**28**(4):327-328. DOI: 10.1089/jop.2011.0209. Epub 2012 Feb 3

[40] Nekoukar Z, Zakariaei Z, Taghizadeh F, et al. Methanol poisoning as a new world challenge: A review. Annals of Medicine Surgery (London). 2021;**66**:102445. DOI: 10.1016/j. amsu.2021.102445

[41] Pakdel F, Sanjari MS, Naderi A, et al. Erythropoietin in treatment of methanol optic neuropathy. Journal of Neuro- Ophthalmology. 2018;**38**(2):167-171. DOI: 10.1097/WNO.0000000000000614

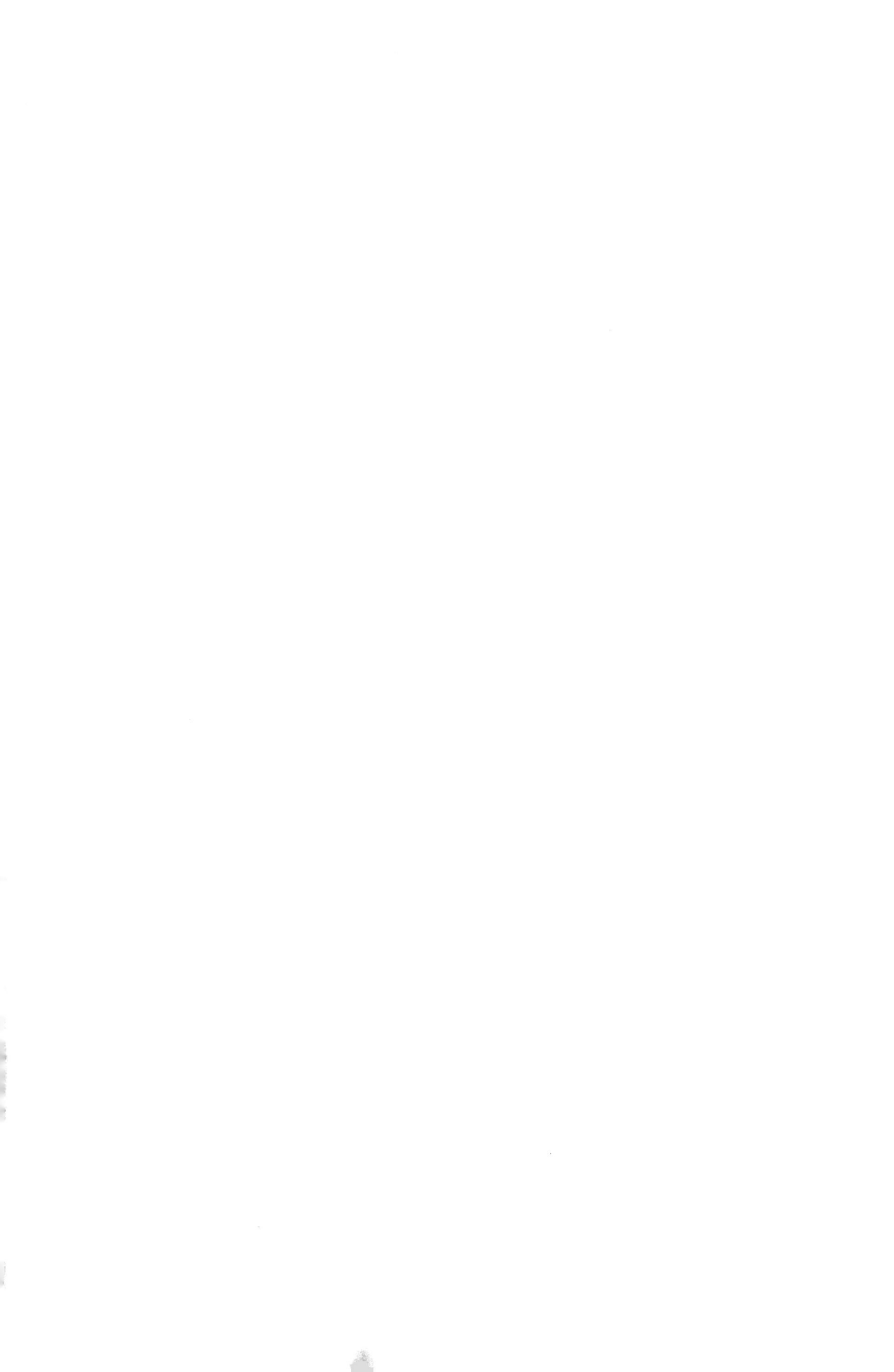